# IT'S NOT A DIET

# IT'S NOT A DIET

## THE NO CRAVINGS, NO WILLPOWER WAY
## TO GET LEAN AND HAPPY FOR GOOD

## DAVINIA TAYLOR

First published in Great Britain in 2021 by Orion Spring
an imprint of The Orion Publishing Group Ltd
Carmelite House, 50 Victoria Embankment
London EC4Y 0DZ

An Hachette UK Company

5 7 9 10 8 6 4

Reviewed for scientific accuracy by
Dr Tamsin Lewis @sportiedoc wellgevity.com

A CIP catalogue record for this book is
available from the British Library.

ISBN (Trade Paperback) 978 1 3987 0342 1
ISBN (eBook) 978 1 3987 0343 8

Printed in Great Britain by Clays Ltd, Elcograf S.p.A.

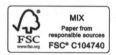

www.orionbooks.co.uk

*To my darling dad for his dopamine and my mum for her perseverance and endurance. Miss you Mummy, wish you could have seen me do something useful at long last!*

# CONTENTS

# INTRODUCTION

# HOW IT ALL BEGAN

When I was thirty-five, my mum died of breast cancer and I hit rock bottom. Deep in grief that was just too big to manage, I didn't know how to deal with the stress I was feeling. I'd long ago given up the excessive drinking that had taken over my twenties, and so I took refuge in food. Lots of it.

I went off the rails and I ate everything I could get my hands on, so, on top of my overwhelming sadness, the weight piled on. My doctor warned me that I was borderline obese. My body was swollen, I felt constantly ill and some days I found it hard to get out of bed. I didn't know how to get myself out of that hole. I knew the way I was living was unhealthy, but I kept putting off getting healthy until the next day. This might sound familiar to you. It's so easy to make those promises that everything will be different tomorrow.

But when tomorrow came, I didn't do anything to help myself because I didn't know how, and most of the time I felt so rubbish about myself I didn't feel like I was worth it. Add in a serious lack of energy, massive sugar cravings and two young sons to look after, and you've (quite literally) got a recipe for disaster.

I tried low-fat and calorie-controlled diets and couldn't stay on them (later I understood why, and I'll explain it to you too). I tried juice diets and diet clubs, but nothing worked. In the end, I got so depressed I ended up throwing money at private doctors in the hope they could 'cure' me. I wasn't even sure what I wanted to be cured of – depression, grief or just a general feeling of being unhealthy and incredibly unhappy. All I knew was that I wanted to feel better. I was put on high doses of bipolar medication, which took the edge off my anxiety, but made me feel ten times more sluggish and zoned out, and even less inclined to eat well and exercise.

Even with the help of medication, I couldn't get out of the negative loop that I was stuck in. My whole body was inflamed, though I didn't know that's what it was at the time. Inflammation is when every single bit of you feels swollen and heavy, like you're trying to move through gel. It's not about body shape because you get slim girls who feel like they're always bloated and in constant pain and feel bulky, and you can get curvier girls who are super-flexible and feel great and are able to exercise really well. If you're inflamed, you will know it because you're exhausted and your muscles hurt, even when you haven't been exercising (and exercising might feel impossible).

I later learned that this bloated, heavy feeling is caused by consuming inflammatory ingredients like sugars and soy and certain highly refined vegetable oils, especially sunflower oil. If you take sunflower oil out of your diet you are going to start losing serious weight fast because it's in practically everything we eat, and it's one of the main causes of inflammation. If only I'd known that back then.

I wasn't exercising because I was too tired even to go for a short walk around the block. When people say, 'Just start with a small walk and build from there', they don't realise how overwhelming even a walk can feel when you have nothing in the tank. I found it was much easier to have a bar of chocolate to feel better, because the sugar gave me an energy hit and a temporary bit of comfort from my intrusive thoughts.

I'd always had a tendency towards self-destruction, and I've never really understood why. Back in my late twenties, I was running with the 'cool' crowd, I had a wardrobe full of nice clothes and I was married with a baby. From the outside, I had everything, but inside, I felt like I was drowning. I was constantly trying to find the answers for questions I couldn't articulate. I felt negative, I felt like a failure, and I couldn't see a way out. I also couldn't understand why I felt that way. I was living a 'fairy-tale' life, so why did it feel like a nightmare?

I had so many years of jetting here and there, going to crazy parties and meeting 'cool' people who should have been on top of the world with all their money and their fame. And honestly, not many of them were.

I was living a majorly hedonistic life back then, but for all the fun I seemed to be having, underneath I was really struggling. I was on a path to self-destruction, and no matter how hard I tried, I couldn't find a way to turn things around. There wasn't any past trauma I could attribute it to, which made me feel even worse. I had a wonderful upbringing, so why couldn't I just be 'happy'? Why wasn't it that simple? I questioned whether it was genetic or hormonal, or whether I was simply a terrible fuck-up of a person. I couldn't understand myself, which made things even more frustrating.

## REHAB WAS JUST THE BEGINNING

I went to rehab a few times for a month here and there in the UK, but I didn't ever stick at it. I always managed to find a way back to my old crew and my old habits.

In the end, my no-nonsense mum forced me into rehab in South Africa in 2009, so I was far away from temptation, without a credit card, a phone or even my passport, all of which were taken away from me.

I was there for twelve weeks and I came out clean and sober and I began trying to turn my life around. I started attending AA meetings and I had to cut ties with people who had been a destructive influence in my life. I knew if I didn't, I would have no chance of staying on the straight and narrow.

I was suffering from the pressures of a divorce, my child being taken away from me and potential financial ruin. And, if I didn't stay clean, potentially dying. It was a no-brainer, really.

But that doesn't mean I sorted everything out for ever. Rehab isn't a one-and-done situation, it's something you're engaged in for the rest of your life. That makes it sound like a prison sentence, but it isn't. What you learn in rehab is that the little things you do to take care of yourself really add up to big changes in your physical and mental state.

In some ways what I learned in rehab from alcohol was the start of how I turned my life around from another rock bottom. It didn't happen overnight. It always makes me roll my eyes when people talk about a 'journey', but for me, getting healthy was one! And journeys start with the first step.

Mine began with a bit of running. Nothing like I can do now, but at least I was doing something. I still had a pretty crappy diet, but taking the alcohol away and starting to move my body a bit more made a big difference.

I think because I wasn't constantly feeling dreadful due to hangovers, I became more aware of how certain foods made me feel. I always blamed feeling crap on booze, so when I felt a bit exhausted or hungover and I knew it wasn't down to wine, I started questioning what else it could be.

It's only now that I can look back and see that certain foods actually triggered my cravings for alcohol. In rehab, they recommended that I always have sugar with me, so that if I got a craving for alcohol I could eat some to help it go away. But actually, it was making me want alcohol even more, and later I understood why – and will explain it to you, too.

Even though I'd quit booze and should have been on a high, my satisfaction in life was diminishing instead of increasing because my addictive brain was still searching out things that would make me feel good, like sugar. I'd stepped off the booze merry-go-round, but I'd hopped onto the next one, which was driven by carbs and anything else that could give me an instant 'fix'. For some people that fix is gambling or sex or shopping, but for me it was food, and all the toxins from the processed junk I was eating were limiting my ability to produce serotonin, the happy hormone. So it stands to reason that sometimes I missed that warm feeling of alcohol. I hadn't found alternative healthy ways to feel 'good' at that point.

I had never heard about the gut/brain connection which connects what you eat to how you feel. No one had ever told me, as I later found out, that I was oestrogen dominant and that was affecting my mood. All I got told was that if I put down the booze everything would be OK. But that was only the beginning. I had so much more to learn, and it's taken me years to do it. So many people relapse after getting clean, and I do wonder if it's because we don't learn about healthy ways to feel good. We're not educated about how what we eat affects our mood, and why certain foods will make us fantasise about 'the good old days'. I honestly think that learning about nutrition and exercise is the reason I'm sober today.

Let me just point out here that I am not totally anti-alcohol, and this isn't a book that says you have to be sober to be healthy. I think alcohol is great for some people and they have a good time on it, but in the end, drinking didn't make me sociable and happy, it became so destructive and dangerous.

I spent the next five years after rehab 'white-knuckling' it, which is what they call it in AA when you're staying sober but not thriving. You're just about holding on to life and you haven't worked out what's next for you. I was still out of shape and feeling rubbish and relying on prescription medication. I knew I wasn't going to drink, because that wasn't an option, but everything else was game on. Imagine going through each day trying not to drink but not having anything positive to focus on!

It took me a long time to find the thing that was going to make me feel naturally good, and as it turned out, that thing was the (sort of!) simple act of taking care of myself.

I had to learn how to ditch my destructive old habits and replace them with good ones, but it wasn't an overnight process. I made a lot of mistakes along the way. I listened to so-called 'experts' who were dishing out dodgy nutrition advice, I over-exercised and put my body under too much stress and I had to go back to the beginning and start all over again. Eventually I realised that in order to find out what was going to work for me, I had to do my own research and be my own guinea pig because all of our bodies are individual and they respond to what we put in them and how we treat them in different ways.

## THE BIG TURNAROUND

I was about four years sober when I met my husband Matthew. We've got the same sense of humour and he'd just given up drinking himself, so we were on a similar path, which I think really helped me to get into a good headspace when it came to my health. We were learning bits and pieces together as we went along, and we devoured wellness books and shared things we'd learned about online.

Things started to really change for me when I read a book called *The Diet Myth* by Tim Spector, professor of Genetic Epidemiology at King's College, London, and I learned about bloating and the gut microbiome. I also started thinking about the connection between alcoholism and trauma. That's when my interest in genetics began and, armed with new knowledge, I started piecing things together.

I started counting chemicals in food instead of calories. Whenever I'd gone on a diet previously I'd restricted the number of calories I'd eaten. I'd happily eat three 'diet' biscuits for breakfast but I wouldn't go near an avocado because it was too calorific, and there's no such thing as a low-fat avocado. What I hadn't been aware of is that our bodies can easily process an avocado because it's natural and it contains 'good fats', which I'll discuss in more detail later. But those biscuits? They were packed with chemicals – fake ingredients and inflammatory fats that were making me ill, only I didn't know it. Once I was armed with the information that I needed to remove chemicals and not calories from my diet, my life began to take a different trajectory.

When I got pregnant with my fourth son Jude, I started eating a paleo diet to be healthier, which you'll no doubt have heard of. The paleo way of eating is about getting as close as possible to the diet of our ancestors – cutting out processed food and chemicals, and sticking to meat, fish and vegetables. All of a sudden, I understood how what I ate when I was pregnant could affect the baby's developing gut microbiome, and that what I was putting in my mouth was having a direct effect on him and on me. It was fascinating, and I felt so much better.

After I had Jude, I lost weight quite quickly, because my hormones were more balanced due to my diet. I wasn't actively trying to lose weight, but instead I was trying to work with my body instead of against it for the first time in my life. I stopped seeing my body as the enemy, and started to see how I could understand it, and give it what it had been needing all along. I started to eat so that I would *feel* better, and looking better was the side effect rather than the end goal.

People always want to know, 'How much weight did you lose?' We all love a good before and after story, so I totally get it. I've yo-yoed a lot, but at my heaviest I was around 13 stone. I'm now between 8½ and 9 stone, so overall I think I lost over sixty pounds over the course of several years. I have gone up and down here and there, but I don't often think about numbers like that. What really counts for me is the energy I've found, the enthusiasm for life, the happiness I feel day to day, and how much easier it is to ride the emotional ups and downs that everyone experiences.

## PATIENCE IS A VIRTUE, BUT IF YOU WANT QUICK RESULTS, I PROMISE YOU CAN GET THEM

I would say that it took me about six months before I felt happy in my body, but I promise you can put a serious dent in your fat stores and improve your mood significantly within a week or two by doing the same things I did. In fact, you can alter your mood within forty-eight hours just by removing sugar and refined vegetable oils from your diet, adding in real, natural foods, and going for a walk every day. It can be as simple as that.

I'm not suggesting that everything in my life is somehow magically perfect now, though. My mental health and addiction issues are something I am incredibly open and honest about, and I'm certainly not zen all the time now. I'm human! I have to get four kids to school on time every morning, and I still go crackers if I get a parking ticket. I'm not Gwyneth Paltrow. I'm real, and I say it like it is.

What I learned is that so many of the issues I was facing back then came from trying to pretend I was something I wasn't. We all do this, right? Trying to pretend you're happy and fine, even when you're depressed. Trying to be understanding when you're angry. Let me remind you that you're not a bad person because you're feeling pissed off about something. You are allowed to have feelings. Perfection is a big old myth. Have you ever met anyone who's perfect? Because I certainly haven't.

We all have flaws and we're all trying our best. We all get angry at times, and that's *OK*. I love the fact that there is so much more transparency now due to social media (in between the airbrushed bullshit), because it's helping to normalise being normal!

Everyone has stressors. We all have our own film that is constantly playing in the background, whether we're struggling due to family illness, relationship issues or worrying about our kids.

I have learned that modern stresses – the non-stop news alerts, the family demands, an actual global pandemic! – put us all in fight-or-flight mode. We're on constant high alert, and that makes us stressed, and stress makes us crave ways to chill out – which may be carbs or sugar. (We eat them because they work.) One of the most important ways to begin to turn that around is to learn ways to switch off and give our bodies and minds a chance to recover. If your body is telling you that you need to take a break and relax, go and do it. It's not because you're lazy, it's because you need it. We all need to learn to read the signs and take care of ourselves, because no one else is going to do it for us.

I'm hoping this book is going to show you how. I'm not an expert, except on myself, and I'm not some drill sergeant who is going to tell you that you have to do everything my way or you're a failure. I'm someone who's learned to listen to my body and tried out new ways of looking after myself (some of them really simple, some of them a bit out-there) and what I want is to help you to do the same.

If I could give you one bit of advice right now, it would be to take all the energy you're putting into fad diets and put it into becoming genuinely healthy.

If you're currently on a low-fat diet, you're not taking care of yourself, you're torturing yourself. You're taking something away your body actually needs (don't fear the good fats, which are packed with antioxidants!) and not replacing it with anything helpful, or doing anything to change your mindset.

Cutting out sausage rolls for two weeks will not help you to change your thought patterns long term, and yet you're expecting your body to magically change shape for good. The two have to work together.

You might think that if you lose weight quickly, you're going to feel amazing, but that will only happen if you feel good mentally too. Depriving your body is going to make your brain sad. Then when you inevitably binge again, you'll get a food hangover, and you'll feel even worse.

You have to stop blaming yourself for your cravings and counteract them instead. You need to stop feeding the demon within, and I'll show you how to do that by isolating the things that trigger you and hacking your way around them, otherwise you'll be trapped in this cycle of guilt and shame for ever.

Take it from me, it's not possible to bully yourself into feeling good. Feeling amazing needs to come from a place of *wanting* to feel amazing, and knowing that you deserve it. You need to get your body back in balance after years of dieting.

Come on, you and your body deserve a chance. You cannot exist on air and processed protein bars. Let's stop restricting and eating less, and put more good things in our bodies instead. When have you ever heard anyone say, 'Oh my God, I've put on so much weight because I've been eating too many vegetables'?

I'm not expecting anyone to pick up this book and change their habits overnight. That certainly didn't happen to me. I had to build up to it. If you've had years and years of hopping on and off diets and trying every fad going, the chances are you've probably lost a bit of trust in your body. I know I had. I didn't trust my body not to put on weight when I started eating butter and other good fats, but I had to take a leap of faith because nothing else was bloody working for me.

My two-week reset plan is going to give you a real head start in changing how you think and feel. It takes everything I learned over several years and brings it into a short, sharp reboot for your system, and gets you on a fast track to feeling your best.

Try to keep an open mind as you read on. If what you're doing was working, you wouldn't be reading this book. So give something different a try. You may not love all of the food suggestions I make, but I'm not saying anything unrealistic like 'You have to eat raw beetroot three times a day.' I'm giving you loads of options and scope, so you're bound to find things you like.

You may miss certain foods to start with, and that's normal. I did too. But once you start feeling better, I promise it will be so worth it and you won't want to go back.

On the flip side, you can't expect to buy a book and read it but not do any of the things that are suggested, and then get annoyed when your life/body/mindset don't change. Sadly, it doesn't work like that.

Here's a bit of tough love for you – no one can change your body except you. You can hire people to clean your house and you can employ people to keep your garden in check. You can even hire a personal trainer to help you get in shape, but if you don't turn up for those sessions, nothing is going to change. If you don't physically do that run or those sit-ups or that class, your body and your attitude are going to stay the way they are. It's like someone who wants to quit drinking who buys every bit of quit-lit going, but doesn't think they actually need to give up alcohol as well. No one can do this for you. It's time to take responsibility.

If you've got a plan, you're already halfway there. And now you've got this book, you've got one.

## BIO-*WHAT?*

You'll hear me talking about biohacking in this book, but don't get freaked out. It's not as sciency and geeky as it sounds. (Who I am kidding? It's *totally* geeky. But fun geeky, and really accessible. You're probably already biohacking on a daily basis without even realising it.)

Essentially, biohacking is DIY biology. Biohacking aims to get our bodies into a state of homeostasis, or balance. It's about trying to live as close to the way our ancient ancestors did as possible, to work with the way our bodies have evolved, and to hack our way around the modern overload of toxins and bad foods. We can't go back to hunting and gathering and living in caves – and we don't want to: I'm not giving up my online shopping for anything – but we can learn to give our bodies what they have evolved to need.

Biohacking is about taking back control of your health and brain function using nutrition, lifestyle changes and self-exploration. And, if you want to go *deep*, also using science (it's a rabbit hole you may never find your way out of). I have found that the majority of the biohacking information that is already out there is geared towards men. This book will be for everyone, but it's especially aimed at women who are struggling with weight or hormonal issues, because that's what I've been tackling myself.

I've searched high and low and read everything out there, documenting my journey on Instagram as I go. I've separated the fact from the fiction and the gold from the scrap metal, and I've put it all in this book. I'm a consumer of every health trend out there, and I've experienced a lot of weight issues and depression, so I know what works and what doesn't.

Some people think you have to be rich in order to biohack, but that's absolutely not true. I'm going to give you both high-end and free options, and everything in between. I'm not expecting everyone to run out and buy a cryochamber or join a gym. You've got a shower, so you can do DIY cold therapy in your bathroom, and you've got a living room, so you can work out at home for nothing.

The great thing is, you're probably already biohacking in some way already – you just don't realise you are.

You can take what you want from this book and leave the rest. Some of it will be for you, and some of it may not be. You might be looking for help with PMT, you may want to find an alternative to junk food for your kids, or your husband may want to blast away his belly fat. There is something for everyone.

I'm going to tell you what has helped me to change personally, and then it's all about tailoring it to your own life and finding out what does and doesn't work for *you*, rather than worrying about what everyone else is doing. I am not an expert, and don't have any qualifications in medicine, nutrition or therapy. This book is an account of my personal experience and you should check in with your doctor before taking up my recommendations

Please note, this is *not* a diet book. Diets make you feel crap. This book will make you feel amazing!

# MOOD

If you're anything like me, your mood can change fifty times a day, depending on outside stressors, busyness levels, hormones and *definitely* a crap night's sleep.

All of those things have a massive knock-on effect when it comes to how we act each day.

So often, when these stressors bring us down, we eat crap food because our energy is low. Or we skip exercise because our PMT is telling us we want to hide under a duvet. But I have learned that there are immediate ways to turn your mood and your energy levels around to hack your way into a better mood, no matter what is going on. Once you know these tips and tricks, and understand the science behind them, you'll have enough knowledge to turn every day into one that counts.

The main thing everyone always asks me about having lost weight is, 'So what do you eat?', or 'What *don't* you eat?' And I really get that. It's what I used to ask people too. We'd all like to discover that 'one weird trick that melts fat away' or whatever the latest online clickbait says. But the thing that changed everything for me when I hit rock bottom was paying attention to what was going on in my head first. I was so desperate to feel better I'd have tried anything. Everything else – weight loss, energy, motivation – came from trying to get well in my head first.

So bear with me. We'll get to food, I promise, but first we need to understand where we're starting from. Try not to skip ahead to look for quick-fix tips – we're looking for a sustainable, joyful way to get healthy here, not a crash diet. And that means getting familiar with *why* we feel the way we do about food, exercise and ourselves.

## IT'S TIME TO STOP PUNISHING YOUR BODY, AND START PAYING ATTENTION

I was out of touch with my body for such a long time. I expected far too much from it, and I basically took the piss. I wanted to be able to spend three days partying, and then go to bed for twelve hours and expect to wake up feeling and looking vaguely back to normal. Funnily enough, instead I looked puffy and grey and felt horrific.

Did I then want to make myself a massive salad and a smoothie to offset the damage I'd done? No, I wanted to eat ultra-processed and ultra-palatable food and drink more wine to take the edge off the desperation I felt. Balance was not a word I was on good terms with.

I'd go through spates of looking after myself better and then it would all go horribly wrong, and I'd feel furious that my body was 'letting me down' by gaining weight. I was only in my twenties and I felt like that meant I ought to be naturally thin, no matter how many toxins I stuffed into myself. (I was also hanging around with fashionistas, which didn't do a lot for my self-esteem.)

And then, in my thirties, I was overeating in a way that was so out of touch with what my body needed. I was eating to cope with big emotions: it had nothing to do with hunger or nutrition (a concept I barely understood back then). I felt like I 'deserved' the extra weight, and I was not only depressed, but disgusted with myself for what I saw as my lack of self-control.

I know so many people – men and women – who are out of touch with their bodies. I knew that if I was going to get mine back into a good state, I had to make friends with it first. I know that sounds woo-woo, but I didn't go and dance naked in a forest at moonlight in order to gain more self-acceptance. I just made a really simple decision, and that decision was to look after myself.

After years of massive self-abuse, I finally recognised that I was never going to shame or humiliate or judge myself into a better lifestyle. I'd given it a pretty good go over the years, but it just never worked. Think about it. Would you tell your friend she was a disgusting fat loser with no willpower? And if you did, would you expect that she'd answer, 'I'm so grateful you said that, now I'm going to change my ways and get healthy'? Of course not. She'd be furious with you, and would probably – understandably – feel much worse about herself than before.

Once I had this realisation, I started treating my body with respect and my brain started giving me good feedback. I'm not talking running marathons every morning here. I'm talking going for a ten-minute walk and getting fresh air into my lungs. That's how I started. Slow and steady. And then I built up from there.

What I learned is that if my body is working optimally, my brain is working optimally, and I want more of that amazing feeling. Your body and mind are not two separate things, they work in synergy, and you can't trick one into feeling/looking good if you're not looking after them. They are too clever for that.

So it took a bit of effort to change things. And it wasn't overnight. But I realised I couldn't magically fool my body and my brain into looking after me with no effort on my part. I wasn't going get to get a toned body from sitting around watching box sets, and I wasn't going to get a happy brain if I was putting shit into my body and berating myself all the time.

I had one of those 'I cannot feel like this for-fucking-ever' moments, and that was the catalyst I needed to propel me forward. I had to realise I deserved better, and thank God I did.

As a result, I've gone from being exhausted, bloated and depressed, to healthy, happy and thriving, and I will never, ever go back.

Just to be clear, I haven't magically got the perfect body these days, just because I lost weight. I've got cellulite, I've got stretch marks. My body has had four kids and it's done incredible things. I've put it through hell and I've hated every part of it, but now I respect and embrace it, faults and all.

Everything I'm recommending in this book is safe to try, unless you have underlying health conditions, in which case you need to discuss any changes to your diet and fitness with your doctor. And when it comes to doctors, make sure you do your homework yourself before just trusting what you're told.

As I'll explain in more detail later, many years ago I paid a private doctor a fortune to put me on bipolar medication, even though my instincts were that it wasn't the right thing to do. Then I found a young NHS doctor who really listened to me and proved to be my salvation. If it wasn't for him, I'm not sure I'd be writing this book.

Above all, trust yourself.

## START PAYING ATTENTION

I am passionately anti-diet and I want people to ditch the idea that you need willpower to lose weight or feel good. You don't have to white-knuckle it through some crazy meal plan that you find impossible to stick to. Forget depriving yourself: the first thing you need is a massive dose of self-care.

There will always be temptations when you're changing the way you eat. I'm not about to deny that. For me, sugar and cheap processed carbs are the things I find myself wanting when I'm tired or stressed. But I've learned that they're going to make me feel low, and that will lead me to wanting more sugar and carbs, and then I'll feel worse. Sometimes I eat them anyway – I'm not perfect! And a slice of cake is not a line of cocaine, it's just food. But I remind myself that the goal is always 'Will this make me feel good?', not 'If you eat this, you're a terrible person and a failure.' Notice which one sounds punishing, and which one sounds encouraging.

The first thing I want you to start noticing is how different foods and drinks make you feel, both in your body and in your mind. We are all so used to eating mindlessly, not paying attention to what we're consuming, eating on the go, picking up something pre-prepared and then wondering why we feel lethargic and tired.

So step one is really simple:

**Don't change anything in your diet yet, just start to notice the effect of what you consume.**

For many people, alcohol is a substance whose effects we are used to feeling – especially after overconsumption! We know if we drink too much we'll have a hangover. In my case, I drank so much that I had to give up altogether, and that has taught me a lot.

Since rehab, it's very rare for me to crave alcohol. I think that's probably because I learned so many incredible tools in recovery, I now know that alcohol is not an option for me. It's something I will hopefully never touch again as long as I live, despite it being so readily available. Do I ever miss drinking? Sometimes. Does it ever feel like a good idea? No. I don't crave alcohol when I'm sad and low. It's when I'm happy and the addict in me thinks, 'Let's get even happier'. We're talking holidays, beaches and girls' get togethers.

When I'm down, I've got all kinds of things in my artillery to pick myself up – and I'm going to share them all with you here in this book. I've got exercise, I've got hot and cold therapy, I've got supplements, I've got breathwork, which are all strategies to get me out of a low mood. But it's when I'm happy I think 'Ooh, I want more of this good feeling, where's the wine?' Thankfully, my brain has learned that alcohol is not something that I have in my life, and I've worked really hard to train it that way.

## MOOD DIARY

When it comes to training *your* mind, I'd like you to think about how you're going to track your mood from now on. Start to keep a record of what you eat, how much you move, and how you feel afterwards.

When I started out on this journey, I used to record everything I ate, and how I felt afterwards, in the Notes app on my phone. I found this was the easiest way for me to keep track

– I always had my phone nearby, and I didn't forget what I'd eaten or drunk when I was out and about. You may prefer to keep a notebook or a spreadsheet. Just make sure it's something that you're going to find really easy and simple to fill in every day.

Before you start to change your diet, notice how your body and mind are reacting to the foods you usually eat. Make a note of what you eat, and at what time. Note how you feel immediately afterwards, and how you feel an hour afterwards. We are often so used to feeling bloated or heavy or exhausted that this feels normal to us, when in reality it's a signal that our body is out of balance. In order to really notice the changes we're about to make, we need to have a clear record of where we're starting from.

Also note how much you move, and how this affects how you feel. Again, no need to make dramatic changes at this point, we're just noticing how we feel when we sit on the sofa all day, versus how we feel when we've been out for a walk. Nothing major.

You won't need to keep this mood diary for ever. I don't track this in my Notes app any more, though I have a fitness watch and other trackers. But in the beginning it is so helpful to be able to refer back to your diary to remind yourself, when you fancy scoffing half a packet of biscuits, how you're going to feel afterwards. Or if you are making excuses about why you don't want to exercise, you can have a reminder close at hand about how good you will feel when you've done it.

If, like I had, you've lost touch with what makes you feel good in a sustainable, happy way, rather than a cheap sugar high or alcohol buzz, you're going to need to start really noticing how you feel throughout the day. Our bodies are giving us feedback all the time. We've just all got very good at ignoring it – or being so used to having indigestion, or a low mood, or no energy, that it feels normal to us.

My family and I had a long tradition where we'd have a chippy tea on a Friday night, which is fish, chips, gravy, curry sauce, mushy peas, mashed potato and a sausage on the side. I happily joined in every week because that's just what we did, and I didn't want to be the one to break the tradition.

Every Saturday morning, I felt so weak and terrible and, because I'd started paying attention to my reactions after eating, I knew that meal was to blame. I couldn't escape the awareness that all that food fried in inflammatory oils was crucifying me, but I didn't want to be the one to ruin it for everyone else. But it was no fun for the kids when I didn't have the energy to mess around with them the next day.

Then I learned that if you take activated charcoal tablets they will help rid the body of unwanted substances. The charcoal is made from coconut shells, and when ingested it binds to toxins and chemicals to keep your body from absorbing them. It's such an effective substance it's sometimes used to treat poisonings or drug overdoses in hospitals. It is important to note that activated charcoal will also bind with medication, as well as vitamins and minerals, so please do not take it if you are on medication as it can interfere with its effectiveness. It should be used infrequently.

I started taking activated charcoal after every takeaway or 'bad' meal to try to lessen the damage, and it definitely helped, but I still wanted to nap every Saturday afternoon.

Eventually I had to return to my question, 'Does eating this make me feel good?' And I admitted the answer was no, which meant I had to change it. I started to cook my own healthy version of fish and chips so that I could still feel like a part of the family tradition, but not have the massive comedown afterwards.

So although I had discovered a 'quick fix' with activated charcoal (and I do occasionally still take it if I've overindulged), the real fix was to address the meal that was making me feel unwell.

I care about myself and my body now, and it's taken a long time to get here, and I don't ever want to go back to the bloated, miserable, knackered mess I was. I don't want to be in a processed-cake coma for days on end. As much as anything else, it's so boring.

Now I'm in a place where my body is balanced and I don't crave those cheap dopamine hits you get from sugars. I can have a biscuit (if I really, really want one) and not have to finish the entire packet. I can have a handful of crisps (cooked in olive oil) and not want to eat eight more bags. I genuinely don't want to do that to myself. I don't have a constantly flashing 'fuck it' button any more, and miraculously my cravings for junk food have gone. I'm going to tell you how I hacked my cravings for crap in the food section, so you can do the same. But I only got there by addressing my head first – so keep reading and don't skip ahead!

## CRAVINGS AND ADDICTION

I know some people think I've had it easy because I came from a privileged background (my dad is a very successful businessman). But illness, poor mental health and addiction don't discriminate. I have fought my fair share of battles over the years, from divorce and chronic post-natal depression to alcoholism, grief and extreme weight fluctuations.

Addiction comes in many guises, from alcoholism to gambling, sex, food and prescription drugs (and that's just the tip of the iceberg).

I've got a feeling most of us have got addictive tendencies. I am an extreme person in pretty much everything I do and I've accepted that about myself, but I reckon we've all got some kind of 'ism', whether it's a dependence on being busy or an obsession with our phones. When I look around, I don't see many people that are really fully in tune with themselves.

Our senses are being screamed at every time we walk down a high street. There are fast-food places and coffee shops everywhere and they're all targeting you constantly to keep consuming and 'treating' yourself.

My mate had it drummed into her when she was a kid that McDonald's was not for every day, it was just for a treat, so it became the forbidden fruit. Now when she walks past a branch she's always tempted to go in and have a burger just because *she can*. We're having to deal with those kinds of food triggers every day, and if you haven't built up your nutritional armour, the chances are your brain will say 'fuck it' and will be in there munching on a double cheeseburger quicker than you can say 'Ronald McDonald looks like a nice man' (in my opinion, he's a health hazard).

Your 'treat' may look different from a Big Mac, but we all have that one thing we crave. The thing we tell ourselves at the time that we 'deserve', and then we feel terrible about ourselves afterwards. I find it really helps to identify the story you are telling yourself about your craving. Do you eat or drink because you're sad or lonely or bored? Find the feeling behind the craving and you begin to lessen the craving itself – you see it differently.

Some people respond to trauma and stress better than other people, and find it easier to resist cravings when they're anxious or depressed. Part of that response is genetic, meaning you've inherited your ability to tolerate stresses from your ancestors. But there is some amazing new science about our genes which has transformed our understanding of how we might adapt our own responses to triggers and cravings.

It used to be thought that we inherited our genes from our parents, and those genes largely dictated our health, but recently the science of epigenetics has turned that belief on its head. Epigenetics means 'on top of' genetics – and it's the science of how your behaviours, such as diet and exercise, and your environment, can cause changes which affect how your genes work.

It seems that while our genes themselves are 'fixed' (i.e. you can't change your DNA) the 'expression' of the gene (i.e. how it behaves) can be changed by your lifestyle and environment. So you might have the gene that predisposes you to obesity, for example, and yet never become obese. It's often said that 'genes load the gun, but environment pulls the trigger'. I'm all about pulling the right triggers when it comes to my own genetics, and helping to support my body to resist cravings that will harm my health.

When you find yourself stressed, you may begin to crave eating, drinking or smoking to make yourself feel better. I have found that understanding why these cravings happen can take away some of their power over you.

When stressed, your levels of the hormone cortisol go up. Cortisol is the fight-or-flight hormone, and its purpose is to let you know that you're in danger (even if the danger is just a row with your partner). Rising cortisol triggers a drop in dopamine levels – dopamine is the neurotransmitter that plays a big role in how we feel pleasure. We get a hit of dopamine when we do things that make us feel good. Like seeing our posts being liked on social media, or eating something delicious. It feels good, so you want more of it (that's why one biscuit is never enough). So when you're stressed, and your dopamine drops, it's natural for your body to crave the quickest ways it knows to get that pleasure hit – food, alcohol and even drugs.

Once you can get your head around that chemical response in your body, it's easier to understand why we're driven to do the things we do, and we can remove that nagging self-blame voice. You're not a failure if you experience a craving.

My drug of choice was wine. It gave me a feeling of motivation, happiness, confidence and productivity. But it was a false high, and I always paid for it *big time* afterwards.

While I was in rehab, I asked my counsellor, who was twenty-five years sober, why we keep doing things that we know are bad for us. His reply? 'Because shit stinks, but it's warm.' That saying really resonated with me and I still think about it to this day. We stay stuck in old habits because they're comfortable and it's what we know, even if they're bad for us.

If the only way we know how to feel good in the short term is to indulge in things that actually make us feel bad in the long run, we have to recognise that, and turn it around. We have to begin to see that what was once a 'treat' is now something we may need to change.

Understanding our cravings is how we begin to let go of them.

## HABIT IS HUGE

We're all creatures of habit. When I go to a public toilet I always go to the second one in the row, no matter how many there are. I never go in the first one, but why not?

My friend says the best bit of advice anyone ever gave her was 'always use the first toilet in public loos because it's the one that's used least'. Now I know that I'm going to step out of my comfort zone and experiment with cubicle one!

It's silly little subliminal habits like that which happen without you even realising it. If something as ridiculous as choosing a toilet cubicle can become ingrained in us until it becomes an unconscious pattern, imagine what else can.

Habits are formed when the brain converts a sequence of actions into an automatic routine. Our brains are wired to look for ways to save time and energy, and habits take less effort than learning something new, hence they are so easily ingrained.

A simple trigger sends your brain into auto mode, and it quickly switches into its learned routine. Throw in a reward, like food or a sense of achievement, and you've created a firm habit loop of trigger, routine, reward.

The habit becomes so automatic, your brain isn't even a part of the decision as to whether to do something or not. Think about brushing your teeth – you probably don't have to force yourself to do that every day, it's just something you do without thinking about it. The brain doesn't recognise the difference between good and bad habits – it just recognises the energy-saving shortcut, and does the action automatically. This is why it's essential we recognise our habits ourselves, and make a concerted effort to change the ones that are doing us harm.

It's hard to just stop a habit cold turkey. We often need to replace a habit we're trying to change with something new. For instance, if smokers want to quit, they sometimes replace cigarettes with vaping. Or they may change their route to work so they don't automatically light up at the same place each day.

So if you get up every day and have a sugary tea and a processed breakfast bar, and you've noticed that you have a crash of energy afterwards, before you go into the kitchen try doing five minutes of exercise or some breathwork first. Confuse your brain. You are in charge! Make that new habit.

I'm not saying for a minute you have to give everything up at once. People who have addictive personalities like me will want to change everything in a week because they're all about the high of instant results, but some people will suit taking it more slowly. Keep paying attention and do what works best for you.

Once you've kept your food and mood diary for a week, write down some habits you'd like to change in response to your own personal needs and triggers. These will be different for each person, so I'm not going to dictate what these should be (although later I will be offering advice).

Keep your habits positive and motivating. So rather than saying 'give up sugar' like it's a deprivation, focus on 'have more energy by cutting down on sugar'. And you don't have to do it all at once. If you're reliant on sugar, perhaps cut out sugar in your coffee first, then chocolate and then wine, but do it over the course of a few weeks. Take baby steps.

Here are a few examples to get you started.

**The habit I'm willing to let go of is:**
eating a sugary breakfast each day.

**The habit I'm introducing into my life is:**
walking for twenty minutes every morning.

Go at your own pace. It's not a race. Your body has taken a long time to get here, so it could take a long time to switch things around. Be patient, because you *will* get there. The fact that you're reading these words means you want to make that change. Set yourself motivating goals each week and make it manageable. No one's judging you, and this is your life and no one else's.

## MOOD-BOOSTING HABITS

Once we become aware that the 'treats' we so often reach for in order to feel better often leave us feeling worse in the long run, we may wonder what to turn to instead. Instead of feeling like you're depriving yourself of a treat, try to add in a new treat. Something that won't leave you feeling worse the next day.

Here are a few of my favourite mood boosters to try instead of the usual treats like a glass of wine or a sugary frappuccino.

If you're not sure when you first try these, persevere for a bit. Remember your first taste of alcohol? I bet you found that pretty weird too! Let's get ourselves used to craving something that will boost our mood rather than diminish it.

**Kombucha** If you usually have a glass of wine at the same time every night, try instead a glass of fermented kombucha, which is a delicious sparkling drink full of probiotics and antioxidants. Did you know that most of your serotonin, aka the happy hormone, is made in the gut? So adding in foods that encourage a healthy gut – like probiotics – can improve your mood. And you may find that it's the ceremony of stopping for a drink that relaxes you, rather than the wine itself.

**L-theanine** is an amino acid that's found in both black and green tea leaves, as well as an edible mushroom called Bay Bolete. You can take it in tablet form or as a powder. It chills you out without making you feel tired, and lowers anxiety. It is often taken with coffee to help avoid the jitters that can sometimes come with caffeine.

**Lemon balm** is (funnily enough) a lemon-scented herb that is a part of the mint family. You can make tea from fresh or dried leaves, or you can take it in tablet form (often combined with L-theanine). It's said to boost your mood and help you to de-stress, as well as helping to boost cognitive function.

**GABA** (aka gamma-aminobutyric acid) is a naturally occurring amino acid that is made in the brain and can also be taken in supplement form. It's said to improve mood, reduce anxiety and help with PMT symptoms.

**Reishi coffee** I have found reishi coffee, which is made from the reishi mushroom and contains no caffeine, is a great leveller. I know mushroom coffee sounds weird, but try it. Make yourself a lovely creamy one and feel the day drift away (do I sound a bit like a naff TV advert?).

## ANXIETY AND DEPRESSION

In 2008, after having my eldest son, Grey, I had been put on strong antidepressants by a private doctor I went to see in Harley Street, which, as you can imagine, wasn't cheap. But I was so desperate at the time, I would have done anything to feel better.

He diagnosed me as bipolar. Around that time, bipolar was the buzzword in mental-health issues and it had become 'fashionable' (Kerry Katona and I were like the figureheads for it), so I think it was too easy to put me in that box.

When someone in a white coat tells you you're bipolar and you're holding on to the edge of a cliff by your fingernails, you don't question them, because you just want to feel better. These days, I feel that what he really should have done is look into what my hormones were doing.

I'd had IVF in order to have my first son, Grey, because my ex-husband and I had been trying to have a baby for several years with no luck. I do not remember the IVF specialist telling me I was more likely to get post-natal depression because of the huge change in hormone levels, and all the drugs they pump into you. Personally, I think that should have been a priority, given that I was pretty much crying all day, every day.

When I had a follow-up appointment a few weeks after giving birth, I mentioned how down I was feeling to the IVF specialist and it felt like such a horrible, sordid conversation. I don't think we ever discussed whether it could be a chemical imbalance.

He referred to me in paperwork as 'mother', which was awful in itself. He wrote things like 'mother is having baby blues', 'mother has suicidal tendencies', 'mother has alcohol problems'.

It was all very cold and very Victorian and I thought there must be something seriously wrong with me.

And so obviously it seemed right to me when the next doctor suggested I should be taking hardcore medication every single day. I was on a serious amount of medication for a number of years, and it had got to the point where I didn't know how to strip it back. I was too scared to stop, so I sleepwalked through each day, barely functioning. It wasn't a life, but I was so grateful not to feel suicidal.

I was on SSRIs, which increase serotonin levels and are supposed to make you 'happy', but I can only assume the cocktail of meds I was on were keeping me level and stopping me having the lows, but they also stopped me from having any highs. I had flatlined. Everything was just . . . OK. To try to feel even a bit of joy, I was having sugary Starbucks and fizzy drinks, as well as more stimulating foods. The pay-off was that I was getting more and more unwell.

It was only by chance that I was thrown a lifeline when I moved house. While I was registering with Holland Park Surgery, I had an appointment with this really nice NHS doctor, who looked at my file and said, 'Hold on, what's been going on with you? My God, you're on *serious* bipolar medication and really high doses of antidepressants. What's been going on?'

After I'd explained everything, he told me my story was a classic example of still being medicated for what had been going on ten years previously. He said he thought I'd actually been suffering from post-natal depression all that time ago.

The doctor took me off the medication very slowly over the course of a couple of months, and that was the start of me seeing light at the end of the tunnel. I 'woke up' again, and I didn't feel out of control and reliant on drugs for the first time in so long. Without wanting to sound too dramatic, it's entirely possible he saved my life.

I'd gone from being addicted to alcohol to allowing medication to do the numbing for me, so I'd just switched one addiction for another.

I'd effectively been overdosing on meds for five years, after years of partying and no sleep, and putting huge amounts of strain on my brain and liver, and probably messed up my neurotransmitters in the process.

Neurotransmitters, such as serotonin and dopamine, are the body's chemical messengers that carry and balance signals between neurons, aka nerve cells, and they work constantly to keep our brains working properly so we feel balanced. They're essential for everything from breathing to our heartbeat and our concentration levels, and they can also affect psychological functions like joy, pleasure, fear and mood in general. Basically, we want to keep those bad boys as healthy as possible if we want to feel good.

Thankfully I managed to wean myself off the drugs OK. That was the point where my life began to turn around. I knew there had to be another way to balance my brain chemicals, I just had to find out what it was. I started researching like a madwoman, and when I discovered biohacking, it was like a dark curtain lifted and I could see clearly for the first time in years.

It's really important for me to say here that if you are suffering from depression or anxiety and you're on medication, please, please don't just stop taking it. If you do want to stop, you need to do it really slowly and carefully and with the help of your GP or a specialist.

Please don't chuck the boxes of drugs in the bin and go cold turkey, or load up on supplements and hope for the best. It has to be a slow process that is well monitored. There's no way I could have stopped taking my meds without the help of my GP, so please do get proper help and advice.

## IMMEDIATE ACTION FOR MOOD

As I was weaning myself off the drugs, I began to explore other ways of boosting my mood and there were three steps that made an enormous difference. I still do each of these daily, and if you want to improve your mood immediately, I recommend you start here. This is the most basic form of biohacking – it's free and it's instant.

1 **Cold showers** I know, it sounds a bit mad. But as I was weaning myself off the anti-depressants, I read that cold-water therapy can instantly balance your hormones, and cold showers were a huge help for me. I'll go into more detail later in the book, but you can start by simply turning your shower from hot to cold for ten seconds each day, and then build up to a minute under the cold water.

2 **Cut out inflammatory foods** These are refined sugars, processed foods, refined grains (e.g. flours), alcohol and refined vegetable oils (except for olive oil, coconut oil and avocado oil). These foods cause inflammation in your body and in your brain, which contributes to low mood.

3 **Exercise** This may be the last thing you feel like doing, and I get that. By exercise I just mean a bit more movement than you're used to. You don't need to hire a personal trainer just yet – do what you can. Get outside for a walk. I promise you'll feel better for it.

I would never recommend leaping into anything challenging when you're depressed or anxious, and that's why I've given just three simple steps here. If you're ever feeling really low or suicidal, the NHS are incredible and they're there for you, so please never suffer in silence.

I no longer take any anti-depressants or medication, but that's not to say that people shouldn't take them if they need them. No one should be judging anyone else here, and it's a process.

I'm certainly not saying that the only way to be fit and healthy is to step away from all medication, because we are all different. I just found that the hardcore drugs weren't working for me in the end (possibly because I was on so bloody many!).

Once my head felt clearer, I started looking into *why* what had happened to me happened. I went down every rabbit hole going, and began to understand how our brains and our bodies *really* work. And I've never looked back.

## WHY YOU DON'T NEED WILLPOWER

Have you ever heard of someone saying 'I'm miserable, so I really want an apple'? Neither have I. We always want wine or cake, because our brain is craving that instant dopamine high. Throw guilt into the mix because you feel like you have no willpower, and you've got yourself into an ongoing vicious cycle.

Stop feeling guilty, because the bottom line is that you're set up to fail. You're being force-fed rubbish food and diets subliminally via advertising, marketing and social media. The diet industry wants you to fail so that they can make more money from you, which is why you've been on that hamster wheel of deprivation for so long.

It isn't simply a case of saying 'I'm not going to have biscuits with my tea today.' It's about that magic gut–brain connection, which I'll explain much more about soon, and stopping those cravings. In a nutshell, we know a healthy body equals a healthy mind, and vice versa.

Trying to stop eating rubbish if you're dieting is no different from trying not to drink if you're an alcoholic. Now I'm thirteen years sober, I can look back and see that I needed a crutch to replace alcohol, and as wine wasn't an option post-rehab, I turned to carbs.

If you try to stop anything using just willpower, whether it's food, alcohol or drugs, you will end up relapsing because you need to change the way you think *for good* so that you don't need a crutch at all. Even Alcoholics Anonymous and Narcotics Anonymous advocate meditating to enable you to change your brain composition.

Fuck willpower, quite frankly. In my opinion, anyone who is using willpower to lose weight will fail eventually because ultimately, they haven't changed their mindset or their habits. They're just trying really, really hard *not* to do something, and that is unsustainable.

In my experience, if you're prepared, you don't need willpower. As long as you've got everything in your artillery (as in the right understanding of how your brain and body work) and you're realistic about what's to come and how you're going to handle it, you will be fine. If you do that, you won't need willpower because unless there are truly exceptional circumstances (yes, PMT does count, but I'm even hacking that) your cravings won't appear.

What I've found is that it's not so much that we lack willpower, but that after years of dieting and eating badly, our levels of dopamine, serotonin and oxytocin aren't balanced, which means we're always chasing highs and trying to feel 'happy'. But if you get your neural pathways working at their optimum, you've got a fighting chance of sticking at what you intend to do. Willpower will not work, but the right nutrition, supplementation and knowledge will.

First things first. You're not going to be able to stick to any form of diet or health plan if you're in a nutrition deficit, which most people on traditional weight-loss plans suffer from. Shockingly, around 3 million people in the UK are malnourished, or at risk of malnourishment. That's not because there isn't enough food to go round – although sadly that will certainly be to blame in some cases – it's because we're not eating food that is actually *food*. What do I mean by that? I mean food that doesn't come in a packet or a box, but from a plant or an animal. Food that would be recognisable to our ancestors, who never saw a packet of cheese-flavoured puffs in their lives.

If you're exhausted and miserable from not eating enough or from eating the wrong things, how are you supposed to muster the 'willpower' to ditch the rubbish?

People talk to me about willpower all the time, but I promise you don't need it if you've got the right nutrition and brain chemistry. If you can get those two things in balance, your body doesn't crave anything and therefore you don't have to fight against cravings or force yourself to do crazy diets. You also don't have to force yourself to do exercise, because when your energy is ticking over your body is working at its optimum, so you *want* to work out and feel good.

Take away the idea of willpower, and think about getting into a flow state instead.

# WHAT IS A 'FLOW STATE'?

A flow state is when things come to you easily, like back in the day when you wrote an essay at school and the right words popped into your head and all the sentences made perfect sense and it felt effortless. Or, if writing isn't your thing, perhaps it was when you were drawing or painting or acting in the school play. It's when things just click. For instance, when you're talking to someone and the conversation is so natural you barely even have to think about it. It's a high level of concentration, clear thinking, great ideas and motivation.

Eventually, when you've eaten well for a while and you've learned what exercise you enjoy and what does and doesn't work for your body, living in this flow state becomes second nature.

It takes practice at first, but you will get to the point where you can walk around a supermarket without stopping at the shite aisles. Not because you're forcing yourself to, or because you're resisting temptation, but because you're just not that fussed any more and you've changed the way you think long term. That's the ultimate flow state; when maintaining good habits doesn't feel like an effort.

It takes time and effort to reset your body and mind and get well, but once you do, you're set for life. Once your system is reset and your new, healthier thinking is automatic, you'll stop having that mental wrestle of 'should I, shouldn't I?' Instead, you'll be free.

Are you excited? You should be!

I would also suggest that, on a basic level, if you're getting cravings and wanting to reach for the biscuit tin, you should check in with yourself and go through the 'HALT' steps, which are used a lot in recovery.

**Are you:**

**H**ungry?

**A**ngry?

**L**onely?

**T**ired?

If you answered yes to any of those questions, why is that and what can you do about it? If you're lonely, can you call a friend? If you're tired, can you have a nap? If you're hungry and in nutritional deficit, what is something nice and healthy you can eat that will satiate you? Sprinkle some good-quality salt on a boiled egg and whack that down you and see if it helps. If you're angry, can you go for a run or whack your bed with your kid's cricket bat to get some of your frustration out?

Instead of ignoring your cravings, or battling against them, start to listen to them. Your body knows what it needs. When a pregnant woman craves coal, it usually means that she's missing zinc or iron in her body. If you're craving carbs, something is missing in your body, and it's probably *not* a doughnut. You need to figure out what your brain is telling you.

Carbs aren't the devil. They're also in vegetables, and if you eat organic vegetables you're going to get a ton more vitamins and minerals than taking supplements alone. If you have a carb craving, it could be that you need a really hearty vegetable soup to up your vitamin and mineral levels. Or (and I used to hate people for saying this) you could be thirsty and just need to get some really decent purified water down you.

I personally am not great with knowing when to stop when

I eat certain carbs, so I have some rules I live by. It's the reason I generally only have sourdough at night. If I started eating it at 9 a.m., I can guarantee you by the afternoon I would have eaten loads and I'd lying on the sofa in a carb coma. But if I start it later in the day I have a shorter window to eat it in, and so I know I won't go too crazy. I know my downfalls well enough to know when I need to put in boundaries.

You're your own computer and you've got your own map, especially now you're keeping a food and mood diary. In a lot of ways, you know more about yourself than any expert, you're just not used to listening properly.

Start paying attention to who and what triggers you, whether it's being stuck in traffic or someone shouting at you. Do you instantly reach for carbs or sugar or wine when you're low? What are you *really* wanting? What hole are you trying to fill?

If I'm peckish I'll reach for fat now, rather than sugar, as I have learned that will keep me going for a whole lot longer than a box of Maltesers.

Of course, the only way I know this is because I ate many boxes of Maltesers in the past, and learned from it, so be kind to yourself as you work this stuff out. It's a process, and you're bound to make some mistakes – just see them as opportunities to learn a bit more about your body's needs, instead of something to punish yourself for.

## COULD IT BE CANDIDA?

Are you bloated, depressed, craving white carbs and refined sugar? You could well have a candida overgrowth.

Candida is a form of yeast which is typically found in small amounts in the mouth, intestines, and on the skin. It only becomes problematic once it starts to grow uncontrollably, usually internally, which is when you get symptoms and cravings like the ones I've described above.

Candida overgrowth can be caused by a number of different factors, including a weakened immune system, taking antibiotics (which destroys the good bacteria in your gut) or eating too many refined carbs.

I had a stool sample test done five years ago that showed that I had *serious* candida. I was literally full of it, so I was really bloated, my cravings were out of control, I felt really mad and moody, really tired and really depressed. All classic symptoms of candida overgrowth, which wasn't ideal when I'd only just had Jude, as I was trying to look after a small baby at the time.

If you have candida, you will suffer from terrible cravings, because candida is a yeast that thrives on sugar, and it's so bloody devious it sends messages to your brain to manipulate it into telling you to eat more. I wasn't suffering from thrush, which is a huge indicator that you have candida, so it didn't occur to me until I listened to a podcast about it that it could be the cause of some of my problems.

I spoke to a health expert in America who told me, rather bluntly, that candida basically wants you dead. It's a mouldy parasite that wants to take over the whole body and kill you, and then eat your corpse. (I hope you're not reading this over breakfast.) It makes you depressed and miserable.

The worst thing was that I had to post a frozen poo sample over to the specialist in Iowa to get tested.

I suddenly realised quite late one Friday afternoon that I had to send the sample off that day by express mail, but I spent nearly an hour faffing about with the test.

As soon as the test was completed (I won't go into details) I belted it down Camden High Street, overweight and lactating, to try and seek out the FedEx shop.

I eventually found it and joined a long queue, and when I finally got to the front I said to the lady serving me, 'I need this package to go today, please. It needs to arrive in the USA by urgent mail tomorrow.'

There was a queue of people behind me in the silent shop and *of course* she asked me the question I was dreading: 'What's inside?'

The conversation went like this:

ME: 'It's human biology.'
HER: 'What do you mean?'
ME: 'It's a sample.'
HER: 'A blood sample?'
ME: 'No, another kind of sample.'
HER: 'Urine?'
ME: 'For god's sake, it's poo.'

Once she'd stopped grinning, she explained that it was too late for it to be sent that day and it wouldn't be picked up until Monday morning. The sample becomes unusable if it's not with a lab within a day, so I had go home, store my poo in the freezer all weekend, and then go through the whole rigmarole again on the Monday morning.

Still, my friend who works in A&E said someone once turned up to the front desk with a poo in an ice-cream carton, so it could have worse.

I remember being horrified when the candida specialist told me I would have to give up sugar and carbs completely to try to eliminate the evil fungus from my body.

I remember calling her back up and saying, 'I can't do it. I *need* cakes and chocolate. I need to be able to eat toast with my scrambled egg.' She replied, 'You can't, you'll just make the candida flare up and then you'll never get rid of it. Do you want to feel this terrible for ever?' I let out a feeble, 'No!' and mourned the fact that croissants were off the table for the foreseeable future.

We often think of sugary products as fizzy drinks and chocolate and cakes, but so many ready meals are loaded with sugar, whether it's the real or fake kind.

Certain diet companies offer meals that come in at fewer than 300 calories per pack. Now for a calorie count that low, those meals are either made up of loads of fresh vegetables and lean meat, or they're ultra-processed. Which one do you think is it?

If you're buying a 'diet' low-fat lasagne, the fat that's been taken out will have been replaced by something else to make it taste good, and it's likely to be either sugar or sweetener. And we're not talking a high-quality sweetener such as stevia here, we're talking the cheapest stuff the manufacturers can get their hands on.

What people don't realise is that the reason they're so hungry after one of those diet meals isn't just because it's bloody tiny, it's because the hidden sugars are kicking off their cravings and their candida/brain wants feeding again.

Diet bars are the same. Woo hoo, only 100 calories for a delicious chocolate-covered breakfast bar! That bar is going to leave you starving and craving in about half an hour. Then you'll tell yourself you're allowed something else because you really only had a biscuit for breakfast, and by 11 a.m. you're dipping your hand into the office biscuit tin, or rifling through your cupboards for the kids' sweet stash.

We're being sold a lie. That's all there is to it. If something seems too good to be true, it bloody is. You think you're really being 'good' because you're just having what looks like a ready-cooked chicken breast and some veg for lunch, but that chicken has most likely been cooked with sugar and then glazed to make it look more appetising. I mean, come on, at least doughnuts are upfront about what they are.

## HOW TO MANAGE SUGAR CRAVINGS

My candida specialist recommended that every time I had a craving for sugar, I should take half a teaspoon of powdered glutamine powder, which is an amino acid. You can buy this from health-food shops. It is taken sublingually, which means putting it under your tongue and holding it there for as long as you can. Apparently this helps it to be absorbed faster into your bloodstream. After thirty seconds I'd swallow the powder down with some water, and the craving would pass.

You can try this for any kind of sugar cravings, candida-related or not. This method gets straight into your blood and knocks the craving out fast, and it's perfectly safe. You can't take too much glutamine, and to be honest it tastes so horrible you wouldn't want to.

I found glutamine worked in targeting the nutritional need of the amino acid that I was craving, but it didn't satiate my need for something sweet, because that was such an ingrained habit.

That feeling was still strong at times, so when it kicked in, I made myself a 'fatty' coffee with extra stevia sweetener and a little bit of vanilla extract, and that really helped. My fatty coffee is a version of the famous bulletproof coffee, which I talk about later in the food section.

This is my basic recipe.

## *Fatty coffee*

1 mug of hot coffee (I use organic instant)
2 tablespoons MCT oil
(see recommended suppliers at back of book)
1 drop stevia sweetener
few drops of vanilla extract
A pinch of good quality salt (I choose Maldon or Celtic)

Put all the ingredients in a blender and whizz up until combined. You can add a knob of grass-fed butter to the coffee, too. I don't often do this, but it makes the drink super-creamy and that can help with cravings. Don't fear the fats! I know the salt sounds weird, but trust me on this. It adds minerals, and it also cuts through the fat of the coffee and makes it taste better.

~

I used fatty coffees as an alternative to chocolate or bread to get me through those really difficult first weeks of sugar cravings while my brain tried to catch up with the new normal. I think once you know you can do the first week you feel psychologically stronger, and I noticed that the longer I kept it up, the better I felt, which motivated me to stay off the sweet stuff.

## LIVER FLUSH AND COLONICS

I also went for a series of colonics to try to flush the candida out and cure my sugar cravings, but I wouldn't advise people to have them unless they're ill. People often have colonics thinking they'll make them lose weight or feel loads lighter, but personally I think they should only be used for medical reasons. I've been told by several experts that a colonic will remove the good bacteria from your gut as well as the bad bacteria, and you need to maintain a really good population of healthy bacteria at all times to stay feeling well. If you flush all your good bacteria out, apparently it can take six months to get your gut back into a good state using probiotics and prebiotics, which means some serious work and some investment. Is it really worth it for a potential temporary two- or three-pound weight loss?

In order to deal with the candida, and put a stop to my cravings for sugar, I also put myself on a liver-flush regime, which is not for the faint-hearted, but it was a turning-point for me. It doesn't just work for candida, I found it great for rebalancing me as well.

A liver flush is a good thing to do if you're feeling sluggish and bloated, because it can knock out the cravings immediately. I'm not going to lie: it's brutal. But it works. I did a liver flush for one day a month for seven months, and it gave me a good week without any cravings at all. I advise doing a liver flush the week after your period, as this is the best time hormonally. I felt my mood physically lift each time, and the cravings lifted.

Make sure you check with your doctor before embarking on this. It's not for everyone but it worked for me, so it might be worth a shot.

If you fancy braving a liver flush yourself, the instructions are below. It is hardcore and it involves fasting for an entire day, so make sure you've got the time, space and energy to do it (fair warning: you might get grumpy and shout at your husband/ children/dog). If it works for you, I would recommend doing it once a month, but no more.

## *Liver flush*

You will need:
500 ml pure apple juice (preferably freshly pressed)
8 camomile tea bags
3 tablespoons of medical grade Epsom salts
235 ml olive oil (that's not a typo – it's a lot!)
Four grapefruits, juiced.

**7 a.m.** Drink 500ml of pure apple juice

**7.30 a.m.** Drink 1 cup of camomile tea. Continue drinking camomile tea until 2 p.m. eight cups in total.

**5 p.m.** Take 1 tablespoon of Epsom salts dissolved in a glass of warm water.

**7 p.m.** Take another tablespoon of Epsom salts dissolved in a glass of warm water. (Make sure you're near a loo.)

**10 p.m.** Blend the olive oil with the grapefruit juice until it emulsifies into something that looks a bit like a creamy salad dressing, and drink.

**10.05 p.m.** Go to bed. If you struggle to sleep, you may find a magnesium supplement helpful.

**7 a.m.** Take 1 tablespoon of Epsom salts dissolved in a glass of warm water. Make sure no one else is commandeering the loo. You're going to need it.

Eat normally for the rest of the day.

~

## UNDERSTANDING YOUR GUT

Hippocrates said all disease begins in the gut, and I believe depression does as well. Your gut is often referred to as your second brain, and 90 per cent of serotonin, our happy hormone, is produced in the gut. If your gut is in dysbiosis, which means it's lacking in good bacteria, your brain will be unbalanced and you'll feel less happy. Inflammatory foods cause an inflammatory brain, which has a massive effect on your mood.

You are what you eat, and you *feel* what you eat.

There are one hundred trillion bacteria, viruses and other microbes in the digestive tract, which play a huge role in creating our immune system and energy. They also break food down and are constantly sending signals to our brain, and vice versa. The ratio is 80 per cent of signals going from the gut to the brain, and 20 per cent of signals going from the brain to the gut. So you can see just how important it is to have a healthy gut if you want to have a healthy brain.

What you put in your mouth goes down to your gut and affects your brain, so you need to literally 'feed' your neurotransmitters.

Low levels of good bacteria have been linked with health issues like osteoporosis, IBS, cardiovascular disease, obesity, autoimmune disease, cancer and dementia, so it's not just about mood either.

Always think about feeding your brain rather than your stomach, then you'll find your cravings will go and you will actually be able to enjoy eating well, being healthy and looking after your body much more easily.

Everything starts with the gut. If you build a house you always start with the foundations, otherwise the house will fall down. It's like that with health. Unless you've got a healthy gut, you're going to be constantly trying to dodge a sickness bullet. You cannot maintain good health without having a really happy gut.

Your gut is the root of everything. People forget that everything in our bodies is linked and you can't treat just one part of it and hope the rest will be OK. If the heating isn't working in the basement of your house, it's going to be cold in the attic.

Everything has a knock-on effect. I know of someone who went to their GP and told them they were having flare-ups of symptoms including stomach aches, a sore throat, headaches and sinus problems. The doctor looked at her and said, 'Well, they can't all be linked.' What the hell? Our whole body is linked! My friend ended up getting sent to a stomach specialist, an ear, nose and throat specialist, and was even sent for a brain scan; and these specialists treated each symptom as if it was totally separate from the others.

This is why I rate holistic practitioners, such as functional nutritionists, who look at every single part of the body and work out the root cause so they can treat it and eradicate it, instead of finding a symptom and giving you tablets to mask it.

The NHS are incredible and do magical work, but I really

hope in the future they start taking a more holistic view of things and consider just how essential a healthy gut is in keeping the rest of the body well. They would honestly save millions. In Germany they hand out probiotics to patients every time they have to take antibiotics. How amazing is that? Why are we not doing that, or at least suggesting to patients that they buy their own to minimise the damage antibiotics do to our guts?

However, you can take all the probiotics in the world and they won't help unless you're eating well at the same time. Probiotics won't be able to be absorbed properly if there's no goodness for them to attach to, so you'll be paying out a lot of money and getting very little benefit. It has to be a two-pronged attack.

## Help your microbes

Professor Tim Spector – professor of genetics and author of three brilliant books – explains that a healthy gut is absolutely crucial to having a healthy immune system. Gut microbes are so essential that our immune system can't function without them. The human immune system develops in the first few hours after we're born, and each gut microbiome sends out signals to ensure our immune system isn't reacting too much, or not enough.

Research shows that people who have allergies, whether that's hay fever or food allergies, have abnormal gut microbe profiles. Some of that will be down to their immune system reacting badly to the allergy and creating problems in the gut, or it can be that their abnormal gut microbes are predisposing them to allergies.

Either way, your gut microbes have an impact on your

allergies. In studies in Tim's lab he found a situation where a pair of twins were coeliac, but each reacted differently to gluten because they had different gut microbiomes.

Tim explains in *Spoon Fed* that your gut microbes like having a rest in order to function well. If we snack all the time, our microbes don't get a chance to have a break. Later on, we'll be looking at how intermittent fasting can help us feel better both physically and emotionally.

The aim of building a healthy microbiome is to build up as many healthy microbes as you can by eating a diverse range of foods, so your gut and immune system are strong.

While we may not agree on everything, Tim Spector's views on gut health have influenced me. The top recommendations are:

- Increase your intake of gut-friendly fermented foods, like kefir, kombucha, kimchi, sauerkraut, miso and yoghurt

- Eat more vegetables and salads (Tim aims for a variety of up to thirty different plants a week which includes herbs, seeds, nuts and spices)

- Eat good-quality virgin olive oil.

## Beat the bloat

I have always suffered from bloating and I still do sometimes. These are a few things that have helped me get my gut back to normal, and expert Pippa Campbell has more advice below.

**Bone broth:** Bone broth, known to our mums as 'stock', is a liquid made from boiling up – you guessed it – bones. You can buy this from supermarkets, but it's incredibly easy to make it yourself, using leftover bones from your roast dinner. Just add the bones to a large pot with a tablespoonful of apple cider vinegar. The apple cider vinegar will draw out the nutrition from the bone marrow and the bones, and from the connective tissue. Fill the pot with water, and simmer gently for up to eight hours. A good bone broth will cool to a jelly-like consistency thanks to all the nourishing collagen and gelatin that has been released from the bones. Both collagen and gelatin are known to be extremely soothing and healing to the gut as they help to repair the lining of the intestinal wall, and reduce inflammation.

**Molkosan and aloe vera:** An elderly Indian gentleman told me about combining Molkosan and aloe-vera juice to combat bloating. Molkosan is a liquid made from whey, a by-product of the cheese-making process. It is rich in lactic acid, which is known to support the growth of good gut bacteria. I find it invaluable for keeping my gut in optimum condition. I have three capfuls of Molkosan and five capfuls of aloe-vera juice when I wake up each morning. When I first started doing that, I noticed a difference in my bloating within a week.

**Colostrum** is a fluid that is produced by female mammals after they give birth, and it's packed with immune, growth and tissue-repair ingredients. I ended up with really bad gut issues about five years after I gave up drinking, so I can't even blame it on alcohol. It was purely down to me eating what I thought were healthy foods, like lots of sugar-packed smoothies and refined grains, and I was bloated and uncomfortable. Colostrum capsules were recommended to me by a doctor, and along with taking bone broth and collagen, they seemed to heal my gut. I still take colostrum if I feel like I need to, but the difference is that now if I eat something inflammatory (like a pizza) I only look two months pregnant instead of like I'm about to give birth.

**Bovine collagen** is incredible for your gut. It is made from boiling bones to release the collagen protein, which is then usually turned into a taste-free powder. I have it most days, mixed in with water and soluble vitamin C. It's important to ensure that you take a high-quality bovine collagen without additives and from animals that have not been fed hormones and antibiotics.

## Gut health with Pippa Campbell

If you follow me on Instagram, you'll be familiar with the amazing Pippa Campbell (@pippacampbell_health), who is a functional nutritionist, owner of her own lifestyle company and all-round gut guru. I caught up with her to discuss bloating, bad bacteria and IBS (among other things!). Of course, you should always check with a doctor if you've noticed changes in your body.

### ? *What are the main causes of bloating?*

Bloating can be caused by so many different things. One thing is missing good gut bacteria, or the presence of bad bacteria. There's a real tendency for people to bowl in and start taking probiotics, but that can actually make things worse. It can cause an explosion effect, or they won't do anything because the bad bacteria will just gobble it, so sadly it's a waste of money. The wrong food may also cause bloating, and that's why keeping a food diary is so helpful. It can help to unmask what's causing it. You may also be lacking in digestive enzymes, so your food isn't being digested properly. Stress is also a bloating trigger, and breathing really helps with that because it engages the parasympathetic nervous system. I recommend slow breathing, where you breathe in for four seconds, hold for one second and then breathe out for six or eight seconds. Doing that once an hour will make a huge difference.

**?** *How can we find out if we have bad bacteria?*

The chances are you will have symptoms. You may be craving sugar and have wind that has a bad odour. You may feel tired after eating, or get brain fog or an itchy scalp or itchy ears. You can do stool tests to find out. Sometimes I can spot bad bacteria via a consultation and no test is needed because it's so obvious. It's helpful to know what your microbiome is doing so you can target any problems.

**?** *Fermented foods like kimchi, sauerkraut and kombucha are really popular – I'm a huge fan – but are they good for everyone?*

Not everyone gets on with them and the results can be a bit explosive for some people. If you've got candida and you add fermented foods, it can make things worse. The best thing to do is to try them and see if you react. That's the best way to test. So, have a small amount of fermented food on its own, away from other food and drinks and see if you can tolerate it.

**?** *Does alcohol have a big effect on the gut?*

Alcohol depletes your body of vitamins, minerals and nutrients, in particular B vitamins, which are essential for energy, brain function and gut health. It will irritate your gut lining and can have a huge effect on your organs, in particular your liver, and causes damage if you're drinking large amounts. If you're trying to heal your gut, I would avoid it. Alcohol and water are absorbed in the stomach, whereas other nutrients have to pass through your body before you absorb them, so drinking is not ideal if you have any kind of gut issues.

**(?)** *What are the best ways to heal your gut without having to get any tests done?*

Vitamin-D-rich foods, and vitamin-A-rich foods, such as offal, or zinc from seeds and nuts if you're vegan or vegetarian. The most important thing is a varied diet.

**(?)** *Should everyone cut out gluten or do you need to wait until you've had a test done?*

Some people are coeliac, and we can see that in DNA or blood tests. There are also people who are non-coeliac gluten sensitive, for which there isn't necessarily a specific blood test. I think that's where DNA testing can be really useful, because you can see risk factors. If I were to have a consultation with someone, before I do any tests I would check to see if there's a family history of coeliac or other autoimmune diseases. I'd also check whether they had gut symptoms or suffered from IBS-type symptoms. They could then try a gluten-free diet, and if they feel better their body has told them they have issues with gluten without them having to do a test.

**(?)** *Aside from food issues, what are the main causes of constipation?*

An underactive thyroid can cause constipation because everything gets quite sluggish. A lack of bile can also be to blame, so keep an eye on your stools to make sure they're light in colour. That's a sign your gut is working as it should be.

**?** *Can you tell us a bit more about how the magical vagus nerve affects the gut?*

The little-discussed vagus nerve is like a dual carriageway going up and down from your gut to your brain, and vice versa. You know that feeling when you've got to do a presentation and you're really nervous and you get a bit of diarrhoea? That is a prime example of how something going on in the brain and the nerves are affecting your gut. Now imagine how being stressed all the time is going to affect your gut. It's going to have a *huge* impact. That's why relaxation is vital for gut health.

**?** *So many people seem to suffer with irritable bowel syndrome. Has it become a general term for gut issues?*

Yes, I think IBS is just one of these blanket things that doctors say if you have any gut problems, whether it's tummy aches, diarrhoea or constipation. But you have to wonder, what's actually going on? If somebody's been suffering with gut issues for a long time and they've tried eliminating gluten and dairy, they may get referred to a gastro-enterologist who doesn't know enough about diet. These specialists often hand out a low-FODMAP diet, which is supposed to help with symptoms, but there are a lot of foods included that can irritate the gut and cause more bloating, constipation or diarrhoea. Basically, if you get told you have IBS, I would ask for a second opinion.

**?** *I am fascinated by the fact that we've got oestrogen receptors in our gut, which affect our metabolism.*

Yes, we've got oestrogen receptors everywhere. They're all over the body, which is why so many different body systems are affected when we're perimenopausal and menopausal.

Oestrogen will affect serotonin, and a gene called the PEMT gene, which is part of methylation, which means that you then can't make choline, an essential nutrient that is really important for brain health and development. That's why women get brain fog and poor memory. The gut gets affected because 90 per cent of our serotonin resides in the gut.

### ? How can we increase our levels of choline?

Choline is a very important nutrient for brain health, liver detoxification and cell membrane. Things need to get in and out of our cells easily, and if our cells aren't permeable enough they need help with that. You can get choline from eggs and liver, or supplementation with phosphatidylcholine.

### ? Should everybody be taking supplements?

No, not necessarily. We're being told that one of the best supplements to take to prevent COVID-19 is vitamin D. So perhaps everyone should just be taking vitamin D as a preventative measure, especially in winter. Generally, the people who come to see me come because they have health issues, and once we've discovered what's going on with them, supplements can help to get them to a healthy place again. Some people come to me for preventative reasons and I may see a snip on their genes that puts them at high risk of Type 2 diabetes. In cases like that, I will get them to clean up their diet, and maybe take supplements that will protect them. I would never recommend that people start taking supplements without professional advice. Please don't get something because it's advertised on Instagram, makes loads of health claims and the bottle looks nice. You don't always know what you're getting, and they could do more harm than good.

## UNDERSTANDING THE VAGUS NERVE

Pippa mentioned the vagus nerve, and I was interested to know more about this little-known nerve which has such a big impact on how we feel, physically and mentally.

The vagus nerve is a nerve that runs all the way from your brain stem to your colon, so it runs past all your organs and nerve endings. It's responsible for the regulation of your internal organs, so it affects things like heart rate, respiratory rate and digestion.

These days, we use our brains much more than our bodies, engaging with the world online rather than outdoors, and all of this physical inactivity means we're not actually stimulating our nerves in general. If you're not exercising or stretching every day, your vagus nerve is going to get lazy in some places, and it won't fire up properly to connect all of your organs, which could have a knock-on effect on your gut health and your mental health.

If your vagus nerve isn't working properly, you could end up with constipation and inflammation because your gut isn't getting the information that says 'Come on, we've eaten, let's get moving'. And when our gut health is poor, our emotions can be all over the place.

Physical activity is helpful when it comes to keeping the vagus nerve in good health, and so is stress management. Meditating can help to wake the nerve up and tone it, which in turn helps with digestion by telling the digestive tract it needs to move food on. That's why people feel a lot better for doing yoga, Pilates or other forms of stretching exercises. A roller bar is also really helpful for rolling down your spine, and fun stuff like trampolining can help too.

Cold showers also help; I focus cold water at the bottom of my neck when I'm in the shower, which helps to stimulate the vagus nerve. It takes seconds but I do feel like it helps.

## HORMONES AND MOOD

Despite changing my lifestyle, I still have months where I get awful PMT and my mood just crashes. Although I know things like exercise and eating well help hugely, sometimes I have those days where I want to shut myself away with a tub of mini brownies and contemplate the meaning of life. Funnily enough, you can't be that self-indulgent when it's a Sunday morning and you've got four kids and two dogs that all want your attention at the same time.

I love the fact that hormones are being talked about so much more openly now. Things like PMT, perimenopause and the menopause are no longer being whispered about, and I hope the conversation keeps opening up.

I swear that if men had to go through menopause, it would be sorted by now and there would be a really easy way to navigate it. There would be some kind of magic laser that would speed up the process so middle-aged guys could get back to being all manly and shit. I'm not being right-on here, it's truly what I believe.

It's not like menopause has suddenly been sprung on us and it's a big surprise that women have to go through this hell in middle age. We all know it happens to half the population, so why isn't more being done to make it easier? I mean, we can video-call each other on our watches and yet scientists still haven't found a way to make the hormonal transition smoother for women. Don't get me wrong, I bloody love FaceTime, but we need to get our priorities right here.

Having cramps and PMT have become so normal, we don't question them. But we're not actually *supposed* to suffer from pain and mood swings. If we do, it's an indication that something isn't right with our body. The body wasn't designed to feel bad, and pain indicates a hormonal problem that you shouldn't mask by going on the pill, which is what's often suggested by doctors. It's a million times better for you to get to the bottom of what is causing you to feel so bad and address it.

One thing I will say is that we need to be kind to ourselves when we're going through bad hormonal moments. I'm not saying I'm giving you permission to throw down a tub of Rocky Road, but if you're craving bread, go for the best version – which is sourdough, because it can help mitigate inflammation.

Although I know there's a fair amount of evidence that gluten contributes to inflammation, I personally don't advise gluten-free bread because it usually contains sugar. Despite the gluten, you're better off with sourdough because the fermentation process sourdough goes through means it has started to eat the gluten molecules, making it easier to digest. And I prefer white sourdough to brown, because often the husks on the brown loaves make me bloat. Sourdough is how our ancestors would have eaten bread. As with all foods you eat, go for something that's as close to homemade as possible, and stay away from the factory-made foods that are designed with low costs as a priority rather than our health.

If you're feeling really desperate with PMT and you feel like you must have chocolate, I recommend keeping an emergency stash of stevia-sweetened chocolate, because the stevia won't spike your insulin.

I know all too well the temptation to eat junk food around your period, but, if anything, we should eat cleaner than ever around our cycle to support our liver which works hard to flush out all the rubbish we ingest. Energy is stored in the liver, which is one of the many reasons it's so bloody important to look after this precious organ.

Over time it will become second nature to reach for a piece of stevia chocolate instead of belting it down to the corner shop for a giant Yorkie bar. I realise this sounds very simplistic and you may never imagine yourself getting there, especially if you suffer badly with your hormones. But you can, and you will, because your hormonal issues will improve if you follow the advice in this book.

If I have a really bad PMT month, I get a lot of critical inner monologue and I kind of hate myself and give myself a really hard time. I feel 'less than'. I don't get teary, I just get down on myself, demotivated and fearful of the future. Matthew calls it 'beat up Davinia time', and it's so noticeable he can spot it a mile off.

I also bloat and get water retention. The PMT mood swings are far worse for me than any pain I get. There's no point in reading self-help books or trying to talk myself out of it. Inspirational quotes will just make me angry.

I found that my PMT was getting worse over the years and after having a DNA test done, I discovered that I'm genetically predisposed to holding on to oestrogen, especially in the lead-up to my period, which can cause an oestrogen overload and worse PMT symptoms. If your oestrogen goes out of whack, you can get all sorts of horrible feelings, from low self-worth to imminent doom (anyone who suffers from this knows I'm not being dramatic!). Once I had that information, I was able to put things in place and mitigate the symptoms.

## HORMONAL HELPERS

When it comes to hormones, you have to be prepared. If you are a sugar addict you have to attack this the same way I would attack an alcohol craving. If I have a physical craving, I take myself out of the situation. If it's a mental one, I go through the Hungry, Angry, Lonely, Tired list and try to work out what's triggering me.

Understanding your triggers will help you and it will also help those who share their lives with you. This is where your mood diary majorly comes into play. It's such a brilliantly simple and cheap way of isolating the things that send you spiralling and spark off bad behaviours.

Your hormones can trigger cravings, especially for women, depending on where you are in your cycle, so I would also recommend that you get a period-tracking app, to track where you are in your cycle. If you get cravings, you can check in with where you are in terms of ovulation, etc., and maybe get an answer as to why you're feeling this way. There are loads of free ones, or you can pay to have extra features. The one I use is called Flo, and I find it so helpful. I've got friends who are perimenopausal or menopausal, and it's helped them to make sense of things too.

Everyone's hormonal symptoms will be different, so I advise working with an expert before making any major changes to your diet or supplementation, but I've listed below some hormonal helpers which have really helped with my mood swings.

Now, I'm not saying for a minute that taking all of these would work for you because we're all different, I'm just explaining what I had to do personally. If you are planning to take any kind of supplements, I would always recommend getting tests and professional advice. But what I'm trying to demonstrate is that there are options available to you that will help you more than popping two painkillers and opening a bag of chocolate buttons.

**Increase protein and good fats** Protein and good fats help us feel fuller for longer so that we don't crave sugars so much. Upping your protein levels can help with cravings around your period.

**Exercise** For me, this looks like putting on some old-school rave tracks and going out for a long run. That always makes me feel better, even if I often don't want to put on my trainers at first. For you, it might be yoga or something gentler. But moving will always boost your mood, so find what works for you.

**Magnesium** Circulating oestrogen can cause low serotonin levels, so I did some research which suggested my body needed to break down the oestrogen in order to lift my mood. I discovered studies which suggested I could help it to do that by taking magnesium supplements and eating more green, leafy vegetables.

**B vitamin supplement** B vitamins help boost the production of neurotransmitters, helping to keep the brain healthy. B vitamins also balance blood-sugar levels and help stress levels and sleep. I take one 2000ug B-vitamin-complex lozenge at lunch (I don't advise taking these in the evening as I find they can interfere with sleep).

**Folate** I learned that I needed to upgrade my folate by eating more green leafy veg.

**5-Hydroxytryptophan, or 5-HTP** This is an amino acid produced naturally by your body that is converted to serotonin. As a result, it's thought to regulate mood and help with sleep. I find I get a massive mood drop when I don't take 5-HTP regularly. I take 300mg a night before bed so I can help my body manufacture serotonin while I sleep. Please note that 5-HTP can interfere with other medications, so check with your doctor before taking it.

**Tryptophan** This is found in foods like cheese, turkey and sesame seeds, and it may help your mood to increase your intake. In the body it turns into mood-boosting serotonin, melatonin (the sleep hormone) and vitamin B3.

Other vitamins and supplements I have found helpful for my PMT symptoms are listed below.

**Horsetail tea** This gets rid of hormonal water retention, so I'll take it during my period. You can get massive bags of it on Amazon and I find it works a treat. You can also find tablets for water retention in most pharmacies. I don't suffer as much from water retention as I used to because I'm not as inflamed, but it does work really well.

**Maca** This is a dried and powdered root from South America, known for its uplifting and energetic properties. I find it's great to put in my coffee in the morning. You can get it in powder or tablet form, and I stir a teaspoonful into my coffee during the first few days of my cycle.

**Ashwagandha** This is an 'adaptogenic' herb, which means if you're tired it will wake you up, and if you're wired it will calm you down. I find it very calming, so it's great for anxiety and PMT. It's an equilibrium enhancer. I take it whenever I'm stressed, and that's usually when I've got PMT!

**Vitamin D3** This vitamin is amazing for hormone regularity, immunity and heart health. In the summer we produce Vitamin D3 through sunlight on our skin, but in the colder months we are not able to produce enough. I mainly take it in winter.

**Magnesium** This mineral is really calming and great for sleep. I take it as tablets at night, and I sometimes have a magnesium (Epsom salt) bath so I absorb it through my skin.

**Lion's mane** This is a mushroom that looks like a big lion's mane. It's really good for focus and thinking, so it's great if you're going to read a book or meditate. I take it after a workout, and I use a teaspoon of powdered mushroom in a shot of lemon juice.

**Stabilum 200** This is known as the world's oldest supplement and I take four each morning. It contains an extract called Garum Armoricum, which was used by the ancient Celts (third century BC) of Armorica and Ireland to improve resilience to physical and emotional stress. It's great for stressed teenagers who are doing exams, too!

## TWO RECIPES FOR HORMONAL CHOCOLATE CRAVINGS

There are times when only chocolate will do. I get it. The trick is to have the chocolate in a way that isn't going to wreck your mood afterwards. Building in some healthy fats to keep you feeling satiated for longer, and avoiding the sugars that will cause a major energy crash. When I feel a bit 'bleurgh' and hopeless, I'll make myself a huge chocolate avocado mousse with a bit of vanilla stevia in it.

# Chocolate avocado mousse

2 super-ripe avocados
6 medjool dates (remember to take the stones out)
2 heaped tablespoons of cacao powder
half a cup of hazelnut milk
pinch of salt
2 drops of stevia (optional)

Blend everything together in an electric blender, adding more milk if it gets stuck. Don't be frightened of the salt: it brings out the sweetness in the dates. By all means add a few drops of vanilla extract if you want to take it to another level.

I pour the mixture into espresso cups and leave them in the fridge, and generally find they hit the spot during day three of my period. I make these in advance and am comforted by the thought I'm giving my body great nutrition and bioavailable nutrients while getting that feel-good satisfactory chocolate hit at the same time.

~

# Paleo Chocolate Bark

My friend Lucy has created this amazing recipe that you put in the freezer, breaking bits off as and when you need it. It's very rich so it's hard to binge on, but even if you do go a bit over the top, at least you know you're getting good nutrition into your body. Of course it's high in fat and sugar, but your body will be able to metabolise it far better than it will an actual bar of chocolate because the ingredients are natural.

I don't count calories, I count chemicals. I know I will feel satisfied after a bit of this chocolate bark, and it's going to stop me eating several bags of crisps which would probably have a load more calories and zero nutritional benefit.

8 medjool dates (no stones)
1 very ripe avocado
1 tablespoon cacao powder
pinch of salt
splash of almond essence

OPTIONAL TOPPINGS
crushed nuts
edible flowers
chilli flakes
dried fruits

Line a wide baking tray with cling film. Blend the dates, avocado, cacao, salt and almond milk together, adding more almond milk as needed to bring the consistency to that of thick double cream. Pour the blended mixture into your lined baking tray and spread thinly. Top with your preferred toppings. Pop in the freezer overnight, and break open in case of emergency!

~

If all else fails, and you end up eating crap in a hormonal haze, remember this too shall pass. The great thing about PMT is that it has a time scale, and if you can make it through a few days without falling spectacularly off the wagon, you can do it the next month too. Do it in increments and take it one day at a time, and do whatever you can to get your body into a good place so it can carry you through as peacefully as possible (or find a remote place and shout and scream it all out).

## A DEEP DIVE INTO HORMONES WITH DR TAM

I have been working with Dr Tamsin Lewis (@sportiedoc) for a while now, and every time we speak, I learn something new. She consults at The Lanserhof, a medical wellness service in Mayfair. She also runs her own company, Wellgevity, which does deep health screening with a proactive and preventative focus. On top of that, Tamsin is a trained psychiatrist and used to work for The Priory. She also won her first ever Ironman triathlon outright. Phew!

I caught up with her to talk all things hormones.

I find hormones so confusing, and it's only by talking to experts that I've been able to understand them more. I've mentioned that I've always suffered from terrible PMT and while all the things I'm doing health-wise are helping, I really want to learn more about how the hormone system works.

**?** *First off, Dr Tam, why do we suffer from PMT?*
*I hate it so much!*

Achieving hormonal harmony can be really tricky, especially in the stress-filled world we live in. PMT has many drivers. We know how awful some women can feel when our hormone levels start to fluctuate during perimenopause. These fluctuations play havoc with how well your serotonin [the happy hormone] can work. Basically, hormonal chaos!

If you have very low progesterone, or the ratio between oestrogen and progesterone is imbalanced, you can feel anxious or suffer from insomnia. Why this happens can be a combination of genetics, stress, over-exercise, poor diet, PCOS and other factors. If you suffer from PMT, you can benefit from stabilising your blood sugar levels as this impacts serotonin. Eliminate refined carbs and fuel with protein and healthy fats. Exercise is to be encouraged but do not flog yourself. Aim for restorative or low-intensity aerobic activity in the ten days pre-period. Long nature walks!

**?** *Why does PMT get worse as we get older? Why?!*
*I've definitely noticed a difference in my symptoms*
*as I've got older, especially when it comes to low mood.*

PMT symptoms are in part due to a fall in oestrogen. Every time you ovulate, your oestrogen levels surge, and then they drop precipitously over the course of the second half of the month. As we age, PMT can get worse because in some cycles, you may not ovulate, and if you don't ovulate, you don't produce progesterone, our calming, warming hormone. Progesterone converts to allopregnanolone, sensitivity to which is thought to be associated with worse symptoms of PMT and you're more prone to that sensitivity as you age. Our body seems to produce less progesterone as we age for a number of reasons. Largely it's because it's an energy-expensive process and the body gets lazy. Progesterone is our 'chill out' hormone and it activates GABA neurotransmitter receptors in the brain, with a similar effect to alcohol, benzodiazepines and Valium.

**?** *We can take progesterone in the form of HRT to help with our dwindling stores, can't we?*

You can, but the problem is that when some people take progesterone, they don't convert it to this allopregnanolone. But they can convert it down different pathways and some people convert it down pathways that make you feel grumpy and moody. This is known as progesterone intolerance. It can be overcome by using very low doses of progesterone as a pessary (cyclogest) for example, and in some cases compounded lozenges which go directly into the blood stream. Supplements like chasteberry extract, also known as Vitex agnus-castus, and extra magnesium/B6 (25–50mg) and evening primrose oil help.

**?** *And which foods can help? I really try to base what I eat around the time of the month to help ease my symptoms.*

Any foods that boost tryptophan can help because it's an amino acid precursor to serotonin – that happy hormone again! As oestrogen levels fluctuate in this 'luteal phase' you can get more sensitive to lower serotnin levels. There is also a genetic component here. If you're eating foods that boost tryptophan, like dark chocolate, bananas and avocados, then PMT seems to be a bit better. Moderate exercise helps. On the flip side, a high-soy diet can make PMT worse (in Westerners) because they contain xenoestrogens, which mimic the action of oestrogen in the body and can interfere with the usual function of our hormones. I would also avoid heating food or storing warm foods in plastic containers because plastic leaches into the food. When you're drinking takeaway coffee, don't drink it through the plastic lid for the same reason. This is not BPA-related, that's a separate issue.

**Why do we experience changes in our gut and bowel habits when our period is due? I experience gut changes, and I know a lot of my friends do too.**

For the same reason we get constipated in pregnancy: higher progesterone levels, which slow down bowel function. Your body is trying to get you to absorb more nutrients because you might be getting pregnant or you are pregnant at that stage. It basically slows your digestion down so it has more time to absorb nutrients and food. Or that's part of the theory. It has a direct effect on the bowel motility. Also, in the second half of your cycle your womb lining has built up and that is going to cause the release of general inflammatory mediators. That's inflammation in the pelvic region generally, which can have an impact on water retention and that sensation of bloating.

**If you're having a day where you've got hideous PMT, you're tired, you can't function properly and everything feels bloated and awful, are there things you can do to help there and then? Please tell me there are!**

In the acute phase, you can take magnesium, B6 and saffron, which are all calming to the nervous system and help dopamine production. Evening primrose oil and turmeric have also been shown to help with inflammation, and magnesium will also stimulate the bowel a bit to relieve constipation. Celery juice can act as a diuretic, and you can take an anti-inflammatory like ibuprofen (I like Flarin, a liposomal form which doesn't upset the gut). Longer term, chasteberry extract acts as an ovarian adaptogen, which means your body tends to have a higher surge of progesterone, which can improve things naturally. Some people get a lot of benefit from that. Also look at serotonin boosters like 5HTP and Griffonia Extract. Boosting the neurotransmitter Acetylcholine function and dopamine can help, too. Think Alpha GPC 300mg and DMAE 200mg.

❓ *This is something that has always confused me. Why do some women suffer from flu-like symptoms before their period?*

The key word here is inflammation (prostaglandins). Your womb lining is breaking down at that time, so just like when you're preparing to give birth a lot of inflammatory mediators are released. They are similar mediators that are released during flu and infection, so in some sensitive individuals they trigger flu-like symptoms. Anti-inflammatories , like Flarin, bio-available turmeric and essential fatty acids such as DHA and EPA, can also help with that.

❓ *Finally, do hormones in food have a big effect on our own hormones? Surely if a chicken is injected with hormones and then we eat it, we're going to ingest those hormones and that could potentially cause imbalances?*

For sure. Unless we buy organic, the chemicals we ingest get stored in our fat cells and the best way to get rid of those is by sweating, either via exercise or saunas. You can definitely shed some toxins with a regular sauna habit. Ensuring your bowel is regular helps too.

## TESTING, TESTING

One thing I get asked about a lot is what tests people should take in order to make the best decisions for their health. Like I said before, I am not a doctor or an expert, so I can only tell you what worked for me. And I loved the results of a DNA test, which really helped me to understand some things about why I am the way I am. I've done a few different tests, both on online platforms and with Dr Tam and Pippa Campbell, and learned so much. There are lots of different tests available, and some need more self-study than others, so you should have a look around and see which one will suit you best. Or engage with an expert who can explore with you.

DNA testing is so common these days. A simple mouth swab test which you can do from home in seconds. The test isn't affected by supplements or medication. Your DNA is your DNA, so things like HRT or anti-depressants won't have an effect on it (although they can affect what genes are 'expressed' throughout your life – see below).

Once you've got that DNA test, you've got it for life, and you can learn an amazing amount about yourself. If you've got dopamine dominance genes, you could be highly motivated to the point where you burn yourself out. There's actually a gene called the entrepreneur's gene, as many successful CEOs have a particular variation of a certain gene in their DNA, driving their behaviour. That's how powerful genetics can be. Whereas if you are genetically prone to a dopamine deficiency, you're more likely to chase highs, which is where addictive patterns come in.

You can't change your genes but you can change your

epigenetics, which in a nutshell means the way your DNA is expressed. You *can* navigate through and silence 'disease' genes, which is what I've been working on successfully for several years. I cannot tell you the difference it's made to my life.

Just one example. I crave sunlight and I get in a foul mood if I don't get it. When I got my DNA tested, it showed I am predisposed to having low serotonin, which is our happy hormone, so of course I'm going to crave anything that helps boost my serotonin. (It explains my previous issues with alcohol, too.) Knowing that really helped me to understand why I am the way I am.

We judge overweight people terribly, but it could be in part down to their genetics, their environment and their hormones, and they may be craving something that's more physically addictive to them than it is to other people. Some people are genetically predisposed to crave carbs and sugar. I'm not saying that's a get-out, but it is genuinely harder for some people to lose weight than others, and that's because their cravings are so overwhelming they feel they have no choice other than to feed themselves whatever they crave. There are of course ways to stop this!

Professor Tim Spector has done long-term experiments with both identical twins (who have identical genes) and non-identical twins (who don't). Through those studies he's been able to work out whether nature or nurture – genetics or epigenetics – are more powerful influences when it comes to your health. Fascinatingly, he's concluded that it's a draw.

On average, 50 per cent of your traits are genetic, and the rest is down to environment, eating habits and overall health. One identical twin can die from cancer while the other one will continue to be healthy. We are clearly not just our genes.

I like to take the guesswork out of my health, which is why I do tests. It saves time and means I can ensure I'm eating and supplementing in the right way.

I spent years blaming myself for being an alcoholic, feeling depressed and having a low immune system, but testing taught me that so much of it was down to my genes. I also discovered I carry a gene that makes me metabolise carbs, sugar and certain fats slowly, and therefore I put on weight easily.

Since I found out which supplements and foods can help support my weight loss, it's meant keeping my weight at a healthy, stable place is so much easier.

## SHOULD I TAKE SUPPLEMENTS?

I get asked this all the time, and the answer is: it depends. Everyone should check in with their doctor before they start any new kind of regime. The likelihood is that your extremely busy GP may not be that clued-up on functional-nutrition methodology, so you'll need to go in there armed with information. Some doctors are very anti what they perceive to be 'alternative' methods, so if you don't like what they've got to say and they're not helpful, see another doctor.

I'm not dissing mainstream doctors in any way, especially not NHS ones, because they do an incredible job, but most of them don't have the time to sit down and talk to you about natural methods, and neither are they trained to do so. Generally, they have a ten-minute slot, which is enough time to have a quick chat and prescribe you medication. To a certain extent, you have to take control of you own health and work out what does and doesn't work for you. Remember that you know what is normal for your own body, so don't be afraid to ask for a second opinion.

Having said that, a lot of doctors are coming round to a more integrative approach, where they're treating mind and body together. It's going to be a while before a lot of methods that have been previously dismissed by the NHS go mainstream, but I'm comforted when doctor friends assure me things are heading that way.

There are lots of vitamin supplements that supposedly incorporate every vitamin you need in one tablet. I've tried a lot of those, and so far none have done anything for me. I was taking seven of one brand a day at one time (the recommended dose!), and I didn't feel any difference.

It's so easy to spend a fortune on vitamins and, if you're going to take them, you need to go for quality over quantity. There's no point in taking a ton of supplements that aren't going to be absorbed or you're going to wee straight out again. It's easy to read an article and see something on Instagram and think that tablet is going to cure all your ailments or give you a sharper mind or balance your hormones, but the bottom line is that sadly there is no one magic pill. It just doesn't exist. Believe me, I've tried most of them.

I've listed some of the supplements I currently take below, but I adapt my regime according to how I'm feeling and my emotional and nutritional needs, and yours may be very different from mine. All I'm demonstrating here is some of the options that are available.

Please also note (once again!) that I take all of these supplements as a result of advice from trained healthcare professionals, and I would never take any kind of supplement just because someone else recommends it. We all have different needs and one vitamin can work amazingly for one person but actually be detrimental to another.

**B12** Thanks to having a comprehensive gene test, I know I have a mutation in my MTHFR gene, which makes me metabolise vitamin B12 from food slowly and reduces my uptake ability. Because B12 makes red blood cells and keeps the nervous system healthy, lower levels can leave me with lower energy and also make me more susceptible to anxiety and depression (and don't I know it!).

Rather than relying on my dodgy genetics and food assimilation to keep my B12 levels on point, I have B12 shots. These are expert-administered injections, which start at around £30. But you can also take a sublingual form of B12 that gets directly absorbed in the blood instead. I always make sure I have enough lithium in my diet to help me absorb the B12 efficiently, which can be found in foods like fish, tomatoes, mushrooms, cucumbers, kelp and pistachios, and sparkling waters like Vichy Catalan.

**Glutathione** My gene test also showed I had a glitch in my genes which means my body doesn't produce glutathione, our master antioxidant, which helps to fight free radicals and pollution and supports the immune system.

Because I can't create that for myself very well, I go for IVs (where glutathione is administered via a drip) to boost it because I naturally have a higher demand for it. A few years ago, I used to catch every cold the kids had, but now I know it's an issue for me I can do something about it. Now I'm ill less often and much more productive. You can also take a supplement as a cream or a suppository.

**Iron** I have a slight problem with absorbing iron so my practitioner, Pippa Campbell, put me on pork pancreas tablets (I know, they sound horrific, but they don't taste of anything) to aid my iron absorption, which helps with my energy levels.

**Probiotics** I think probiotics are a given because they help to keep your gut healthy and balanced. I prefer to take liquid probiotics, either as supplements or as kombucha. The reason these work so well is because your stomach thinks they're water and allows them to go through, rather than the probiotics getting destroyed by stomach acid, which can happen with food or tablets. I find these liquid probiotics are one of the best ways to populate your gut with beneficial bacteria. I also have them via unpasteurised cheese and raw yoghurt, and organic fruit and veg.

**Zinc** I have a naturally low immune system, so I take zinc daily throughout winter, which helps the immune system fight off bacteria and viruses.

## WHAT ARE AMINO ACIDS?

Amino acids are twenty essential and non-essential compounds that exist in your body to play essential roles, such as the synthesis of hormones and neurotransmitters, and building of proteins. Taking them as a supplement is a natural way to boost mood and energy, hence a lot of athletes use them.

All twenty amino acids are important to keep your body working and growing as it should, building new muscles and tissues, absorbing nutrients and regulating your all-important immune system, but only nine of them are considered essential because your body can't make its own, meaning you have to obtain them through your diet (yet another reason why what you put in your mouth is so important).

Those are (deep breath) histidine, isoleucine, threonine, leucine, methionine, phenylalanine, tryptophan, lysine and valine (I'll be testing you on these later). They can be found in proteins like meat, seafood, eggs and other dairy and poultry. As a result, vegans and some vegetarians can be deficient and may need supplements.

## GET CLUED UP ABOUT
## SUPPLEMENT INGREDIENTS

It isn't a one size fits all with supplements, but you can find out what will help you.

Always check the labels of any supplements you buy. Better-quality supplements will contain better-quality ingredients, it's as simple as that. But confusingly, cost doesn't always guarantee quality, which is why I'm going to tell you which brands I trust and believe in at the back of the book.

Yes, your local supermarket may be doing three for twos on vitamins one week, so it's tempting to stock up and save a few quid, but several bottom-of-the-barrel vitamin tablets could be the equivalent to one really good-quality vitamin, so in the long run it does make sense to spend a little bit more. I'm not saying you have to go for the top tier because, much like cosmetics, you could end up paying for the packaging and marketing.

For instance, some cheap omega-3 oil supplements are made from processed fish and fish livers, which isn't great if you're avoiding processed food in your everyday life, or trying to live more sustainably.

A lot have got anti-caking agents like talcum powder, colourings, fillers, toxic doses, titanium dioxide and E numbers and all sorts of rubbish in them, rather than simply the ingredients you need for health, so check the ingredients carefully before you buy. Who wants to be swallowing talcum powder?

The last thing we want to be doing is putting more chemicals into our bodies when we're trying to heal them. I read that we now have to deal with 1,000 times more toxins via our liver than our ancestors did. And we wonder why our poor livers can't cope! If your liver doesn't work properly, it can throw so many things out, including your hormones. You could be taking supplements to try to balance your hormones, thinking you're helping yourself, but in fact you're pumping your liver full of more ingredients it's having to take time to deal with and process.

The main ingredients to avoid are:

**Hydrogenated oils** because they contain trans fats, which may increase your risk of heart disease.

**Artificial colours** which have links to health issues like depression, ADHD and asthma.

**Titanium dioxide** is used as a pigment. There is some evidence to suggest it could be carcinogenic, meaning it could potentially cause cancer.

**Magnesium stearate** which is a synthetic ingredient that is used as a binder and thickener. Incredibly, it can stop your body being able to absorb the contents of the vitamins.

# GOOD MOOD FOOD

I get asked a lot online about what to eat for better mood and, while I think a holistic, whole-body approach is best for mood, using movement, rest, sunlight etc., I do have some general food tips. The following list is not exhaustive, but I have tried to give the most nutrient-dense and bio-available ingredients I find myself using in our house on a monthly basis.

I suggest adding a few of these ingredients to each meal, chopping and changing them regularly to keep the body guessing and adapting to each ingredient. Studies suggest eating a variety of foods will keep the brain healthy and the body metabolically flexible as it searches to utilise each nutritional ingredient in each meal.

Think how our primal ancestors would have eaten as they roamed, their diet changing with the seasons and their surroundings. So, rather than picking a few ingredients and sticking to them, mix it up, keeping your body and brain active in its search for fuel. I've tried to give plenty of choices below.

In times of stress, or during PMT, see if you can reach for these foods before the milk chocolate!

- Cruciferous vegetables, such as broccoli, cabbage, cauliflower, rocket salad. Great sources of **folate**, which supports the regulation of serotonin, your good mood hormone.

- Clams, grass fed beef, organic liver (yes, pâté is a health food!). Rich in iron – low levels of iron are associated with fatigue and depression.

- Salmon, mackerel, krill oil, avocado, ghee and grass-fed butter, organic cold pressed olive oil. All sources of **Omega-3** oils, including **EPA** which helps with memory and **DHA**, a mood-booster.

- Outdoor bred pork, salmon, peas, asparagus. These will increase your intake of **thiamine**. Studies suggest that thiamine supplementation is associated with mood improvement.

- Beef, free-range chicken thighs, sweet potato, banana, pistachio nuts. Adding these to your diet will boost your intake of **Vitamin B6**. Studies show that correcting low levels of vitamin B6 is associated with better mood and increased confidence.

- Cocoa, dark chocolate, mackerel, salmon, halibut, spinach, Swiss chard, almonds, pumpkin seeds, flaxseeds. Sources of **magnesium**, which helps with relaxation and muscle tension.

- Coconut water (unsweetened), avocado, raw organic dairy, wild Atlantic fish, apricots, bananas. Eating these foods will increase your **potassium** levels. Potassium deficiency has been linked to mental fatigue.

- Brazil nuts, organ meats (liver, kidneys, heart etc.), wild fish, outdoor-bred pork. All great sources of **selenium**. Reports suggest that low levels of selenium are associated with low mood.

- Clams, beef liver, raw or organic full-fat milk, butter, eggs, oysters, trout. These are sources of **vitamin B12**, an essential vitamin for humans, which is primarily found in animal products (vegans must supplement with a high quality B12 daily). Reported to boost energy and mood, and to reduce depression.

- Guava, kiwi fruit, strawberries, oranges, broccoli, peas. These all provide **vitamin C**, which has been associated with reducing anxiety and depression.

- Oysters, crab, lobster, clams, shiitake mushroom, lentils (soak overnight before cooking). Good sources of **zinc**, which has been shown to decrease depressive symptoms, as well as support the immune system.

- Organic beef liver, eggs, organic full-fat dairy, broccoli, cauliflower. These will increase your intake of **choline**. Low levels of choline are associated with mood disorders and low energy.

- Eggs, salmon, organic full-fat dairy. Sources of **vitamin D**, which is also made by the body in reaction to sunlight. In the Northern Hemisphere we are often deficient in vitamin D during the winter, and low levels of vitamin D have been associated with depression.

## DAVINIA'S FIVE MOOD TAKEAWAYS

- Keep a mood diary, and track how you feel after food and exercise
- Get rid of inflammatory foods – sugars and refined vegetable oils
- Make at least one new healthy habit that you can stick to every day
- Add gut-supporting foods to your diet
- Track your monthly cycle and work with your body's needs.

# FOOD

I get so many messages on Instagram about what people 'should' or 'shouldn't' be eating, or whether particular foods are 'healthy' or 'unhealthy'. I get asked for daily food diaries and recipes, what to buy, when to eat and when *not* to eat. What all these messages tell me is that when it comes to food, people are *confused*. Big time. And so was I, not so long ago.

My intention with this part of the book is not to dictate to you exactly how and what to eat. I'm not going to say that if you fall off my 'plan' you're doomed or weak. (I'm certainly not immune to falling face first into the kids' leftover chocolates occasionally.) Instead, the goal is to give you the information to make the right choices for yourself with confidence. To see the food you eat as a delicious and joyful way to support your health, not as a punishment for past excesses.

I have learned how eating in tune with my body's needs, and as close to nature as possible, has helped me lose that panicky feeling around food. I now trust myself and my hard-earned knowledge more than I trust the often bogus health claims on a food packet.

My food philosophy in one sentence is this: eat your food as close to its natural state as possible.

So that's an organic chicken leg rather than a chicken nugget. A boiled potato rather than a frozen potato waffle. A piece of an outdoor-reared pig rather than a Percy Pig. Yes, there's a bit more to it than that, or this section of the book would be pretty short! But in essence, that is what I return to and what I suggest you return to when the next diet fad comes along.

I've learned the long and hard way that reaching a healthy weight is not as simple as eating less, and it's *definitely* not about eating so-called 'diet foods' and hoping the pounds drop off. If anything, that kind of yo-yo dieting could leave you heavier than ever – it definitely did that for me.

In this section I'm going to explain why real food, self-care and avoiding marketing diet-traps are the key to long-term, sustainable weight loss.

## WHY I HATE FAD DIETS

Here's something that I know to be true: diets make you feel shit, but eating well and looking after your body does the opposite. I just wish it hadn't taken me over twenty-five years to realise.

My mum raised me in the 1980s on a low-fat diet, which was what experts said was best back then. We were told that 'fat makes you fat' so a generation threw out the butter and embraced low-fat spreads made with inflammatory refined oils. And we got rid of the traditional 'meat and two veg' in favour of low-fat foods that were, unknown to us, full of sugar. My mother wasn't feeding me cakes and sweets all the time – she believed I had a healthy diet – but those low-fat yogurts and pasta sauces meant I became addicted to a high-sugar diet full of processed foods. There was hardly any fat in my diet, which plays havoc with your hormones and keeps you feeling constantly hungry.

Even though my mother had grown up poor and I grew up in an affluent home, my mother would have eaten a much better diet than I did as a child, because there was hardly any processed food around then, and very little sugar.

In my mother's naivety, and because of the low-fat phenomenon, she unwittingly gave me a really bad nutritional start in life. The foods she gave me were bad for my gut microbiome, my hormones, and for my satiety.

My friend's gran used to say to her 'it's not fat that makes you fat, it's sugar', and that's going back years and years. So people knew this a long time ago, it's not news. But then the big food companies came in and marketed sugar at us and we fell in love.

People say 'I don't have sugar in my diet' while they're eating a croissant and drinking a glass of orange juice. Both of those are just sugar bombs. I can understand how having an organic orange is good for you, with all the fibre and vitamins, but not twenty of them squeezed into one glass.

In my twenties and early thirties, my go-to comfort food was always a pizza with mushrooms and onions. I loved Chinese food and I was big on MSG, aka monosodium glutamate, a common food additive that enhances the flavour of food, and has also been linked to asthma and headaches. Obviously once I'd had that, I'd be in a cycle of sugar, salt, sugar, salt. So chocolate, crisps, chocolate, crisps. Just your typical 90s diet. Plus Diet Coke, obviously, because that was 'healthy'.

Then the American market hit and Domino's started sponsoring cool Friday-night TV shows, and all of a sudden we were eating pizzas that were twice the size of the ones we were used to. What no one tells you is that these cheap processed carbohydrates and plastic cheeses make you feel depressed as fuck the next day. I always used to blame booze, but these days I understand that I probably had a food *and* wine hangover.

My weight fluctuated a lot during my twenties and thirties. When I came out of rehab, I was told by a specialist to have sugar as a replacement for alcohol. I started piling on the pounds because I was eating sugar when I would have been drinking. I ballooned and then I got really down on myself because again I felt really inflamed and vulnerable, so I decided to lose 21 pounds in 21 days. I had the most horrific green juices and beetroot juices. I did lose a lot of weight, but not surprisingly it soon went back on again – and the pounds bought some extra friends with them. It's a problem functional nutritionist Pippa Campbell sees in her clinic time and time again.

'With a lot of fad diets, you're severely restricting calories, so quite often you're going into starvation mode,' Pippa explains. 'You lose a lot of water and probably a lot of muscle, but no fat. And as soon as people go back to eating normally, they literally put all the weight back on. Thousands of years ago, when food was scarce in winter and it was a threat to survival, our bodies stored fat. Each time you go on a crash diet, you're storing more and more fat. That then messes with leptin levels, which is our satiety hormone and makes us feel full. When our tummy is full it should send a signal to the brain to let it know we can stop eating, but it stops doing that. That's why people feel so hungry and want to eat all the time when they come off diets. The only way you can get your leptin back into the habit of telling your brain when you've had enough food is by eating the right protein and getting good-quality sleep.'

In a nutshell, if you're doing fad diets, someone, somewhere is making a lot of money from that business model, but it's unlikely you're going to lose weight long term. Someone's making a profit off the back of your misery. Don't get sucked in.

## INFLAMMATORY FOODS

There are certain foods, like sugar and refined vegetable oils, that are known to cause inflammation in the body, and inflammation can contribute towards a number of diseases, including diabetes and obesity. If you want to begin your health journey as soon as possible, the best thing you can do is remove those two ingredients from your diet immediately.

Sugar is bad, but I think refined vegetable oils, which are oils derived from plants and are found in everything from margarine to salad dressings, are worse. I think the body can deal with sugar more easily that it can inflammatory veg oils. I noticed a massive difference in my 'leanness' within two weeks after cutting out vegetable oil. It really makes me retain water, and probably fat too. I'm all for eliminating it completely from our diet.

It's not until you clean up your diet and remove alcohol that you start to notice just how much crap foods affect you. I love the fact that I can now feel what does and doesn't work for my body. As soon as I have vegetable oils, I notice that my mood drops, because my body is so much more sensitive to it these days. Personally, I think that's a great thing, because I have an incentive to stay away from the ingredients that make me feel like crap.

If you have an intolerance to dairy or gluten, your body is

also going to react to those foods. That's why I suggest keeping a food diary, or giving up gluten, dairy or sugar for a month and seeing how you feel when you don't have it, and when you then reintroduce it. There's no point in quitting everything at once because you won't know what's causing your issues.

Take out one thing at a time. If you notice you feel better and have more energy, there's a high chance it's inflaming you.

I've got one friend who isn't overweight, but she said to me she always felt like she was wearing a fat suit. She's a size ten to twelve, but she didn't feel able to wear the clothes that she'd like to because, as she put it, she felt like she was wearing an extra layer of padding.

As soon as I explained to her that it might not be body fat but was more than likely inflammation due to eating things that weren't agreeing with her body, she had a food-intolerance test done (as a birthday present from her husband – what could be a better gift?).

Once she got her results back, she cut out the foods that were flagged up as being particularly inflammatory to her, as well as replacing sugar with stevia, and her entire body calmed down. She didn't 'diet' and she was still enjoying loads of foods she loved and felt satisfied, but her clothes fitted better and she no longer had the dreaded waist/jeans overhang.

## WHY SUGAR ISN'T SWEET

So why is sugar so bad for you? In my opinion, the sugar and processed-food industries are there to make money. Their priorities are profit margins, not the health of their customers. And it is in their interests to create products that always leave us wanting more. The more we eat, the better their bottom line. There is even a word for those processed foods that you can't stop eating – hyperpalatable. These foods are specifically designed to make it hard to stop. It's not because you're weak-willed or greedy.

Sugar in any form is said to be eight times more addictive than cocaine, so it's no wonder we love it so much. But *surely* we all want to be energised and free from cravings? We don't want to be constantly chasing a high. Look at kids when you load them up with sugar. They go mad for a few hours, run around like nutters and then they crash and have meltdowns. We're no different as adults. We are, after all, just big kids, and our bodies work in the same way. If you're pumping yourself full of sugar to give you energy, that energy is going to be so short-lived.

And we all know that the more sugar we eat, the more sugar we crave. So how do we get off the rollercoaster?

During my fascinating chat with Jessie Inchauspe, better known on Instagram as @glucosegoddess, she explained that the more all over the place your glucose levels are, the more likely you are to suffer from sleepiness, cravings, acne, weight gain, a poor immune system, hormonal issues like PCOS and wrinkles.

High glucose makes your body go on the defensive due to all the dangerous free radicals (unstable atoms that can damage cells and cause ill health) which can harm your DNA and cause mutations. As a result, our body uses our vitamin C stores (vitamin C is a rich antioxidant that helps produce collagen, which we know helps to keep our skin wrinkle-free) to fight the free radicals and maintain cellular health. Yes, our bodies sensibly choose our health over our vanity. In other words, the more sugar you eat, the more wrinkles you get.

There was a study done on teenage boys that showed the ones with steadier glucose levels had fewer spots, so it's also likely to have a link with acne.

If your glucose spikes are *very* deregulated, you can even develop Type 2 diabetes and heart disease, as well as increasing your risk of cancer and Alzheimer's. That really shocked me.

In simple terms, we really want to keep our glucose levels as stable as we can. I don't like exercising after eating, but Jessie explained that if you exercise after eating something really sweet, your muscles will contract and suck up the glucose that's in your blood stream and use it for energy. So if you eat a bar of chocolate, do some sit-ups or squats!

When we have a glucose spike, which begins to rise around ten to fifteen minutes after eating and peaks after an hour, our bodies panic at the imbalance. This sends insulin to transport the glucose to our liver and fat cells like a little ambulance, to stop our body being harmed by the excess glucose. If you gain weight from having too much glucose, it's just your body trying to protect you.

Our brains run on sugar, so when our sugar levels crash around two hours after we've had sugar, the body panics and makes us crave more. Hence, we can never stop at one biscuit. Or, if we start our meal with bread and butter, we'll be looking for a dessert. During the dips, our bodies think we've run out of energy and we're starving, so we crave high-calorie foods.

As you've probably already gathered, I like to have my cake and eat it, and sometimes (hello, PMT) I do massively crave sugar, and sometimes I'll give in. If you are going to indulge in sugary treats, Jessie advises not eating them on an empty stomach. Eat some protein or fibre first, which will slow down how quickly your body will gobble up the sugar. In other words, where possible you should have dessert after your meal, rather than sugary snacks in between.

Also, apple cider vinegar is your friend. If you have one tablespoon in a glass of water before you eat something sweet, research by the Diabetes Research and Clinical Practice in 2017 showed that 'Vinegar consumption can attenuate postprandial glucose and insulin responses.' Which, put simply, means that the vinegar can lessen the effects sugar has on our bodies, so it will hugely reduce the glucose spike. Apple cider vinegar slows down the absorption of the sugar and keeps your blood-sugar levels steadier. But avoid cider-vinegar tablets because, ironically, they often have sugar in them.

The order in which you eat your food also has an impact on your glucose levels. If you eat protein or fibre before you eat starches like potatoes or pasta, you'll cut your glucose spike by up to a third.

The worst foods for glucose spikes are the ones that turn to sugar quickest, because glucose is sugar. Starches like potatoes, pasta, rice and anything made from flour are the worst. Starch is basically millions of miniscule glucose molecules attached together, and when we eat starch they get set free in our stomachs and become glucose again. But if I have my beloved sourdough with a source of protein like peanut butter or ham, I'm going to keep my glucose levels steadier.

Sadly, even a lot of the fruits we eat, especially dried fruits, are what Jessie describes as 'sugar bombs'. Tropical fruits like bananas, mangoes and papayas are the worst, not surprisingly, as they're the sweetest, but eating fruit and any other sugars after protein *will* help to mitigate your body's response, and lower the inflammatory response (of course it inflames you too!). A great tip is to have fat like almond butter with your fruit. It tastes bloody great, too.

If you really want to know what's going on with your glucose levels, you can hire a glucose monitor for a couple of weeks for around £40, which will tell you what your levels are doing when. I've worn one and it's proved invaluable for finding out what foods affect my levels the most.

Some sweeteners also spike glucose, so don't think that you're fine using these instead of sugar. I only have Nick's Vanilla Stevia if possible, or @gallybird do drops which I add to coffee.

**Avoid foods which seriously spike glucose**

- Any sugar
- Corn
- Fruit
- Any starch – so pasta, bread, rice and anything made with flour
- Cocktails
- Beer

**The most glucose-friendly alcohol (because I'm not a monster!)**

- Champagne
- Wine
- Spirits on their own, or mixed with a sugar-free tonic water like @gallybird, or soda and lemon

**Galacto-what? Beware hidden sugars**

Sugar is like a celebrity that's trying to hide by having loads of different pseudonyms. He's a master of disguise, and this is a list of all the different names sugar goes under when it's listed on ingredients labels.

When you pick up that 'health' bar and don't see sugar in the ingredient list, don't be fooled. If any of these words are on the packet, there's sugar inside.

## Basic sugars

- Lactose
- Galactose
- Glucose
- Dextrose
- Fructose
- Sucrose
- Maltose

## Solid/granulated sugars

- Sugar (granulated/table)
- Caster sugar
- Coconut sugar
- Demerara sugar
- Dextrin
- Brown sugar
- Cane juice crystals
- Cane sugar
- Powdered sugar
- Crystalline fructose
- Date sugar
- Corn syrup solids
- Muscovado sugar
- Raw sugar
- Panela sugar
- Beet sugar
- Diastatic malt
- Ethyl maltol
- Florida crystals
- Golden sugar
- Glucose syrup solids
- Grape sugar
- Yellow sugar
- Icing sugar
- Maltodextrin
- Sucanat
- Turbinado sugar

**Liquid sugars/syrups**

- Fruit juice
- Evaporated cane juice
- Caramel
- Agave Nectar/Syrup
- Brown rice syrup
- Buttered sugar/ buttercream
- Carob syrup
- Corn syrup
- Barley malt
- Blackstrap molasses
- Fruit juice concentrate
- High-Fructose Corn Syrup (HFCS)
- Honey
- Refiner's syrup
- Invert sugar
- Malt syrup
- Maple syrup
- Molasses
- Rice syrup
- Golden syrup
- Sorghum syrup
- Treacle

## DON'T FEAR THE FATS

Back in the 80s and 90s, fat was the enemy, and I did what I was told by avoiding it. The result was that I was always hungry because my blood-sugar levels were up and down like a rollercoaster. I'd eat a low-fat yoghurt and get high off the sugar, but there was no fat to balance it out and make me feel satiated. It was torture.

Now I understand that fat is necessary, not just for our body's needs and functions, but for us to feel full and to prevent cravings. I can see how my cravings were driven by the very low-fat 'health' foods I was being encouraged to eat.

When you're dieting, you're constantly waiting for the next meal and berating yourself for being hungry. It takes over your whole mind and it's all-consuming.

You can't wait until lunchtime so you can have your Ryvita with low-fat cottage cheese, and then by early afternoon you're starving again and your brain is telling you how weak you are. Instead of feeling satisfied you're constantly spiking your insulin, which makes you hungrier than ever. But if you don't know and understand that, you think you're greedy. After 100 diets fail, you start to think: *It must be your fault, you fat loser.*

Once I got myself out of the diet mindset, I realised it was all about implementing things that were going to benefit me, rather than starving myself and making myself unwell. But it took me a long time to get there. I hope my advice can help you take several shortcuts.

When I began to understand the importance of protein and fats, I understood how I had been depriving my brain by filling my body with hollow diet foods that didn't bring anything to the party. The only thing they were doing was making me feel less hungry, but they weren't 'feeding' me on a functional level. If anything, all the additives were taking goodness out of my body rather than putting any in.

More than 60 per cent of our brain is fat, so it makes sense that we need to consume fat to keep it working well. We literally need to feed our brain. In addition, we need protein to help our bodies repair cells and create new ones, as well as to fuel our energy and transport oxygen around in our blood.

My first piece of advice is to throw away all low-fat foods, right now. Fat is necessary for the optimum functioning of your body and it's time to bring it back into your diet.

However, not all fats are created equal and I have learned that the hard way. So here's my guide to the good, the bad and the ugly when it comes to dietary fats.

## THE GOOD FATS

### Stable fats

These contain a higher ratio of saturated fatty acids and they're best for medium- and high-heat cooking.

- Butter
- Ghee (clarified butter)
- Duck and goose fat
- Chicken fat
- Pork lard
- Beef tallow
- Sustainably sourced red palm oil
- Coconut oil

(The last two are plant-based)

When it comes to oils, always go for cold-pressed or extra virgin oils from organic sources (no GMO, thanks!). Stay away from industrialised oils that are processed at high heat, and those that have been turned into trans fats, which are harmful to health.

### Monounsaturated oils

These contain a higher ratio of monounsaturated oils, which are healthy oils that can help with weight loss, decrease inflammation and reduce the risk of heart disease. They are best used cold or on a very low heat, and should always be kept in opaque glass bottles to preserve them for longer.

- Avocado oil
- Olive oil
- Hazelnut oil
- Macadamia oil
- Almond oil

## Polyunsaturated oils

These contain a higher ratio of polyunsaturated fats, which include omega-3 and omega-6 fatty acids; essential fatty acids the body needs for cell growth, brain function and heart health. They should always be stored in an opaque glass bottle in the fridge to protect the oil from sunlight, which can degrade the quality of the oil.

- Sesame oil
- Walnut oil
- Rice bran oil
- Flax-seed oil

## THE BAD FATS

These kinds of industrialised oils go through high heat processing, and are high in omega-6 which can produce the dreaded inflammation. I suggest avoiding these as much as possible. Be aware that a lot of restaurant food and processed food is full of these oils. Always read the labels, and avoid deep-fried foods where possible.

- Soybean oil
- Canola oil
- Corn oil
- Vegetable oil
- Grapeseed oil
- Safflower oils
- Sunflower oil
- Sesame oil
- Peanut oil
- Palm kernel oil
- Vegetable oil spreads
- Cottonseed oil

(Sesame and peanut oil can be used in small quantities in dressings if they're cold-pressed and organic.)

## THE REALLY UGLY FATS

In my opinion, these oils are so chemical-based they barely even count as food.

- Margarine (urgh!)
- Vegetable shortening
- Partially hydrogenated or hydrogenated oil
- High stearic or stearic-rich fat

## ALWAYS READ THE LABEL

Sunflower oil is my number-one enemy. When will food companies stop polluting our food with inflammatory oils that were originally intended to clean farmyard machinery?

Sunflower oil is so processed and inflammatory, but it's in virtually every packaged food on supermarket shelves, and it's often presented as healthy. Even so-called health experts use it in their products. It's shocking.

Next time you buy a 'health' bar or an energy ball from a well-known influencer or brand, scan the back for the ingredients and I promise you will be shocked at how many of them use oils that are on my banned list, for so many reasons. Believe it or not, sunflower oil, which contains PUFAs (polyunsaturated fats), could actually be worse for your body than sugar. So that's goodbye to margarine straight away.

After doing twenty years of tests, the food industry has finally said that sugar is bad for us, and I think sunflower oil and other fats will be the next thing we hear about.

They have such an instant, inflammatory effect on me. I took one of the kids out to a theme park last year and we were having loads of fun. Then at lunchtime we sat down and shared a bag of chips, because that's what you do at a fun park, and both of us instantly flatlined. I realised they had been fried in refined vegetable oils.

I was supposed to be full of energy and excited going on rides, and all I wanted to do was sit on a bench and laze. My son was affected but not as badly, and I think that's because he doesn't eat as cleanly as I do. My body has become really sensitive to shit.

I wouldn't go as far as to say that it ruined the day, but I certainly didn't enjoy the afternoon as much as I had done the morning. That is the norm for a lot of people. They eat those kinds of foods every day and they don't realise they're ill because it's become normal to feel tired and sluggish. I know because I was one of them.

I look at kids now and I really worry about what kind of state their guts are going to be in when they're older because processed food is cheaper and more easily available than ever.

## Count chemicals, not calories

One of the most important steps in how I changed the way I eat was beginning to understand that it was more important to reduce the chemicals I was ingesting than the calories. What do I mean by this? Well, if you pick up a packet of grass-fed butter and take a look at the ingredients, you'll see two ingredients: cream and salt. If you look at the label on a tub of margarine, that ingredients list is so long! And full of ingredients you'd never find in your home, such as partly hydrogenated soybean oil, vegetable mono and diglycerides, potassium sorbate, citric acid, artificial flavours and palminate.

I realised that the chemicals in these supposedly healthy foods were actually contributing to my inflammation, damaging my liver, my gut and my brain. I was overburdening my system with chemicals it was never designed to process.

My advice, as I've mentioned above and you'll see shortly, is to eat your food as close to its natural state as possible, and read the label. Even better, buy foods that don't need labels on them.

## Increase your protein intake

There is some fascinating new research that suggests that humans and other animals have an inbuilt need for a certain proportion of protein in our diets, and we will continue eating until we reach it, even if that means eating too much food overall.

So if we eat a lot of bread or pasta or other foods that are low in protein, our body will keep us eating in search of protein. But if we eat protein first, we will be less hungry for other foods, and less likely to snack.

We have more than 10,000 proteins in our bodies, in our muscles, bones, tissues, skin and even our hair, and protein also helps to keep our immune system working well.

A lack of protein can lead to muscle weakness, a slow metabolism and even anaemia, and from a diet point of view, it will help you to feel fuller for longer. Because your body has to use more calories to digest and make use of calories in protein, it also increases fat burning and boosts your metabolism.

I have found that eating protein and fat at every meal is essential for keeping me fuller for longer. For me, protein usually comes in the form of meat or seafood, but you can also use cheese, nuts, seeds and beans if you are a vegetarian.

## EATING THE PALEO WAY

Food is such an emotional thing, and for years my self-worth and self-esteem were completely reliant on what, and how much, I ate on a daily basis. I would quantify 'good' and 'bad' days according to what I'd put in my mouth. After so many years spent torturing myself, I knew there had to be a better way.

Because my mum, Lynne, died of breast cancer in 2013, my husband Matthew and I started looking into ways to look after our own health. I started reading so many books about nutrition; I literally couldn't get through them fast enough, and I learned so much. Some of the information was conflicting so I did my own deep research online or by talking to experts, and I basically gave everything a go. I guess I've tried everything so you don't have to!

In my research I learned that, as humans, if we didn't eat fat or protein, we would die, because they are essential to the body. But it turns out there are no essential carbohydrates. So I decided that I would try to go down the route of giving my body what it needed. And that meant plenty of protein and good fats, and minimal carbs, which our bodies can struggle to digest.

The paleo diet was becoming popular around that time, and when I read up on it, it made the most sense to me. It advocates following a similar diet to Neanderthal man, who didn't have loads of grains because it would have taken ages to harvest them as this was before the dawn of agriculture. They also wouldn't have had sugar, because that wasn't introduced to the UK until the eleventh century, but they would have occasionally eaten things like honey and fruit.

In essence, the paleo diet means eating as naturally as possible, and as close to what the Neanderthals would have eaten – so anything that ran, flew, swam or grew.

I read a book that explained how we all started getting more ill and fatter around the time we started using highly refined oils and grains and sugar back in the 1950s, and I just 'got' it. No matter how pretty a food packet looks with a nice cow munching on grass in a meadow, my eyes were opened to the fact that the packet probably came out of a factory and contained umpteen ingredients. That's when I began counting chemicals and not calories.

Because I discovered that most things that come in a packet or box from your local supermarket are processed and will contain sugar and vegetable oils, I knew had to move away from that as soon as possible. I also wanted to avoid the hormones and industrial feeds that are given to factory-farmed animals, in favour of animals that have been raised with higher welfare standards. I started off by eating a lot of organic meat and vegetables, but that's not to say I didn't make mistakes.

One day I bunged some sausages under the grill and then when I looked at the ingredients list I saw that they contained wheat and sugar and all sorts of other things I'd never heard of. I assumed sausages were pure pig, but I started reading packets and picking them apart and educating myself about what was added to the things I ate.

I got obsessed with labels, but not in the same way as I used to be when it was all about the calorie and fat content. I just didn't have it in me, and I had stopped believing all the lies I'd been told for years and years. Instead, I only looked at the ingredients to check for inflammatory oils, or sugars that had been sneaked in under a different name.

I got totally carried away and I felt so passionate about eating completely naturally I had visions of myself making my own bread and organic mayonnaise – neither of which have happened yet, by the way. Then I pulled things back and started to investigate what was readily available that would make my transition into paleo as easy as possible.

A few clicks online and I was lost in a world of paleo bread and all these amazing products that I didn't even know existed. It made me realise that I wasn't going to live a life of misery if I followed a paleo diet. I could still eat amazing food, but everything would be good for my body.

There is no way I could be strict enough to never enjoy anything sweet again, so I researched the best way to still enjoy sweet things every now and again, and discovered that I could, and I wouldn't have to spend days feeling guilty afterwards.

I'm not on a keto diet, which bans all types of sugar, and if I have something that's sweet and considered a sugar, it's a natural sugar. Over generations our bodies have registered what honey is and what a date is. It thinks 'I've got this. It's got some enzymes and antibacterial properties in it. I'll take the good stuff and get rid of the rest.' It uses the good ingredients, whereas even if you have organic brown sugar, your body doesn't understand how to process it, and it will store it for you to wear on the beach.

I do like sweet things, but I'll have the best raw honey on the best sourdough I can find with the best grass-fed butter, and I know that every single ingredient in there has a use, and that's the Paleolithic way of life. You're eating for medicinal purposes.

In a funny way I was lucky, because once I realised how much I'd been conned by the food industry for so long, I got this massive wave of anger and 'fuck you'. It's a catch-22 and all these weight-loss brands use addictive ingredients that kept me going back to their crap foods time and time again. That really fired me up, and rather than feeling despondent about starting another diet that was no doubt doomed to fail, I had faith that I had found a way to change my lifestyle for good. This wasn't going to be another six-month yo-yo nightmare, this way of eating was easy enough to implement into my everyday life, and my health was going to improve as a result.

I found myself talking to strangers in the supermarket like a lunatic about all the terrible ingredients that are in food. I needed to get it off my chest! That's why I turned to Instagram to get the message out. I was so annoyed that we were all being taken for a ride. We were all paying a premium to be overweight and unhealthy. And we were paying twice. Once with our cash and once with our guts and our brains. What the hell? I felt like I'd uncovered this incredible secret I wanted to share with the world.

When I missed things like crisps, I thought about the MD of the crisp company sailing around on his superyacht getting a massage while he ate lobster, off the back of selling the public rubbish, addictive foods, and it made me even more determined not to line the pockets of people who are making us a nation of overweight zombies with vegetable-oil-induced brain fog.

I am so grateful for the fact that I finally woke up and realised that, just like I could never just have one glass of wine, I wasn't someone who could have one packet of crisps and then walk away. It would be a gateway into a bacon sandwich on thick white bread followed by a massive bar of chocolate, and then whatever else was in the cupboards.

The paleo diet allows me to eat really lovely food that I really like anyway, like steaks and roast chicken with vegetables, but I'm never going to go off the rails and eat ten chickens afterwards. The food on the plan leaves you feeling satisfied, not craving more.

Did I have the odd day where I motored my way through a massive bag of Kettle Chips and then searched the cupboards for more? Come on, I'm human. It didn't all fall into place overnight. But did that happen often? Absolutely not. In fact, over time my body became more and more sensitive to dodgy ingredients, so they became less and less enjoyable.

Of course I missed sugar at first because my body was so used to having it, which is why I reached for the glutamine powder when I felt a craving coming on. I also gave myself permission to have bananas in smoothies so I could get that sweet hit as naturally as possible. I didn't go totally sugar-free in the purest sense, but at least a smoothie has a hell of a lot fewer chemicals than a Mars bar, and my body can process it a lot more easily, plus I mixed it with a lot of greens.

Looking back, the one thing I wish I'd known when I first started paleo is that some packaged paleo foods still contain sunflower oil. I felt like I'd been conned when I found that out. I think that held me back and made my mood dip. That was another good lesson in reading labels. You think if you're buying a paleo product the due diligence is done, but that's not always the case. A food can be labelled as paleo and still contain crap.

I would say it took me about a week to get into my stride with paleo. I'd think to myself: *Would they have done this in a cave?* And if the answer was no, I didn't do it. Paleo is basically everything pre-agriculture. I'm not quite full caveman because I still eat sourdough, but it's prepared in an ancient way. I probably eat like people did a thousand years ago.

If I was going to be super-strict, as some paleo eaters are, I would stick to foods that suit my genetic make-up, which is Northern European. But I've tasted the delights of the Far East and I'm not going to spend the rest of my days not being able to enjoy the odd Friday-night takeaway with my family.

I love spices and herbs and fruits and nuts, and I love getting chicken thighs and covering them in Middle Eastern spices and whacking them in the oven. Put them on a bed of rice which you've boiled in bone broth and you've got a great meal. It's not strictly paleo, but I'm doing the best I can and I've tailored it to my lifestyle. And if I have a bit of dark chocolate afterwards some nights, the world isn't going to stop spinning.

My appetite has naturally diminished over time because I'm no longer craving junk, and if I do eat something that isn't great, I know how to navigate my way around it. I'm never going to be that Instagrammer who pretends they live life like a really healthy nun. I don't and I never will, but at least I know the best things to do when I slip up.

## WHY I EAT NOSE TO TAIL

Personally, I feel that meat gives me the nutrition I need to be a good mother, a good wife, and feel good about myself. I need B vitamins. I am descended from hunter gatherers, and we hunted and we foraged and we ran and we swam in cold water. That's how we survived plague, famine and attack. We didn't eat tofu, we didn't eat soy and we didn't eat corn. We didn't have vegan sausage rolls made from the most disgusting ingredients. We didn't have The Impossible Burger that is crafted from God knows what. These foods are made in a lab.

We had steak, we had offal and we had high-density nutrition. That's what kept us strong and healthy and able to wake up every morning alert and ready to take on whatever was thrown at us.

I do try to eat 'nose to tail', i.e. every bit of the animal I can, and use as much of the animal as possible in cooking, so as little as possible is wasted.

I think we were designed to get most of our nutrition from organ meats. If you watch a predator kill an animal, the first things it goes for are the organs. It doesn't go for the thighs or breast like we do. And in ancient societies, the organ meat was highly prized.

Some people are very funny about offal, and I get that. I say give things a go, even if you need to build up to it. I had some chicken hearts the other day that were delicious. They tasted more like mushrooms than anything. If you hate the idea of offal and just can't face it, you can get it in tablet form instead and get the benefits that way.

If you're not squeamish, the cheapest way to eat more meat is to buy the organic cuts that nobody wants and prepare it yourself. Often those bits will simply get chucked away, which is criminal, so they can definitely be picked up for a lot less than you might think.

If you're happy to use offal in your cooking, you can make amazing pâté with heart, liver and lungs – the whole shebang – and have it on some sourdough. People sometimes look scared when I mention pâté because it's traditionally seen as indulgent and fattening, but the fat is where the nutrition is.

I know some people will find my views at odds with the current plant-based movement, but veganism and vegetarianism are not always healthy. I tried to go vegetarian once but I ended up really bloated and lethargic. It just wasn't for me. I was also really peckish all the time and I found my cravings were quite bad. I got really bad wind and IBS, and I put on weight from eating a lot of carbs. I am not genetically predisposed to suit that diet, and when it comes to digesting and taking energy from my food, meat and I seem to be a match made in food heaven.

If you are vegan or vegetarian that is totally up to you. I love animals and if it goes against your beliefs to have animal products in your diet, that is your choice. But it's very easy to be an unhealthy non-meat eater.

There are some really bad vegan foods out there. You can be vegan and live on chips and Oreos (yep, they're vegan, so how do they make them taste like milk and chocolate? What's actually *in* them?). I suggest you ask yourself once again, how close is this food to nature? The more processed it is, the less healthy it is for you.

A vegan diet can be missing a lot of vitamins and it's super-expensive to supplement. You'd need a lot of supplements. It's easy for people on vegan or vegetarian diets to become deficient in iron, B12 and vitamin A, which are mainly found in meat products. Those deficiencies can affect neurotransmitters – the brain chemicals that support mental health.

Let's start eating real food again. If you *are* vegan, eat loads of avocados and turn them into an amazing mousse, and load up on pulses and organic veg – avoid fake foods, in whatever form they come. Ironically, some plant milks are among the most ultra-processed foods out there. Unless you make them yourself, they are full of sugars and inflammatory oils – yet we are encouraged to see them as health foods.

## THE DIFFERENCE BETWEEN ORGANIC AND NON-ORGANIC

I know there are a lot of people out there who think organic food is an expensive indulgence that most people can't afford. But my research has taught me that organic food is worth the extra expense. The main differences between organic and non-organic foods is how they're farmed. Organic fruit and vegetables are grown in much better-quality soil so they will have a higher nutritional content. It's better for every cell in your body.

Also, on a very basic level, it will taste better. You can taste the difference between an organic and non-organic strawberry straight away.

There are no chemicals used when organic food is grown or harvested, whereas non-organic food will have been made using pesticides and weedkiller, while the animals will have been bulked up with corn and other preservatives. Organic is (shocker!) better for the planet, because we're not pumping all kinds of harmful chemicals into our soil.

Personally, even though it costs more, I think organic food is better value because you'll hit your nutritional goals so much faster. You would have to eat a lot more non-organic food to get the same level of nutrients. It will also help with cravings, because your body will feel full and satisfied quicker: you only need to eat one carrot instead of four. You need to eat less because it's so much more satisfying.

If you do buy non-organic fruit and vegetables, you can wash them in baking soda and apple cider vinegar to remove pesticides. Believe it or not, a salad that's covered in pesticides could end up being more inflammatory than cake.

At the end of the day, it's still better to eat non-organic than not to eat any fresh food at all. Real food is better than any supplements.

I give my kids a lot high-fat food, like the meatier cuts of organic beef, which is often cheaper when it's fattier. But that's where all the nutrition is. If you buy non-organic meat, stay away from the fat because that's where the toxins, hormones and crap it's been fed are stored, but if you buy organic meat, keep the fat because that's where the nutrition and the fibre are. If you have the choice between a lean fillet steak for £12, or a rump that's full of fat for about £6 that's organic, go for the fattier organic cut every time.

Chicken thighs are brilliant but they're fatty, so only buy the organic ones. If you buy non-organic chicken, go for a breast, which won't have fat on it, so that cuts down on toxins.

In my humble opinion, regenerative farming is a real solution to our environmental problem. The aim is to restore soils that have been ruined by pesticides and other chemicals, so we can grow even more natural, organic food. We need to go back to basics and feed soil nutrition from farm-animal poo.

I don't agree with factory farming, where people are farming nutritionally negligible livestock in cramped indoor spaces. They are fed utter rubbish and kept in terrible conditions so that meat and other animal products can be produced as quickly and cheaply as possible. It is cruel, and the produce is poor quality. I wouldn't eat it myself or give it to my kids.

You need to look out for the Soil Association on meat labels to know the animals have been reared well. Any organic meat cuts will have more flavour and nutrition. People are buzzing about nitrate-free bacon, which is bacon that hasn't been cured with potentially harmful sodium nitrates, but it's still factory farmed, so I would always go for bacon from outdoor-reared pigs.

Always check the meat percentages on sausages, burgers, meatballs and pies. You want to look for a meat percentage that is over 85% – the higher the better. Watch out for fillers such as grains (like wheat) and sugars (under different names). Also make sure they don't contain vegetable oils: again, check under different names.

I always buy organic free-range eggs because I've discovered that just 'free range' doesn't mean they're all living their best lives. You see 'barn' stamped on a lot of egg boxes, but it's important to understand modern farming methods – a barn is not a lovely countryside outbuilding that's like something out of a kids' story book, it's an industrial-size metal unit where thousands of birds are being fed cheap corn and grains.

Infection is also rife in those kinds of conditions, so it's likely the birds will be pumped full of antibiotics, and potentially growth hormones, both of which we'll ingest if we eat their eggs or meat.

A chicken that has lived life with access to the outdoors, foraging for worms and insects, will lay eggs with a bright orange yolk, which will have more nutrients. Be wary of eggs with pale yellow yolks as these are often a sign that the chicken that laid them had an indoor life.

Corn-fed chicken is now being sold to us as healthy, but that corn is likely to be GMO (genetically modified organism). Chickens are not vegetarian and their flesh should not be bright yellow! In the wild they forage for worms in nutrient-dense soil, rather than pecking grains out of a tub.

Free range is much kinder to the animal, which is so important, but just because they're roaming outside that doesn't mean they're not being fed GMO corn. If they are fed an organic diet, it means they are free to roam and eat worms, like they bloody should!

I avoid farmed fish because it can be harmful to the environment and the fish are more susceptible to infections and antibiotic intervention. Instead, I buy wild-caught fish from the Atlantic.

Prawns from the Far East are generally farmed in boxes and have antibiotics pumped into them, so stay as local as possible. (Scottish fish is brilliant.) Don't be afraid to ask your fishmonger for advice, and always check out the freezer section where fish is often cheaper (but always check the labels!).

I only buy Soil Association organic or EU Organic goods,

because they tick every box when it comes to animals being reared, fed and housed well.

We are being tricked by labelling all the time, so don't be fooled by meaningless things like pretty pictures of livestock or tractors or outdoor scenes. If a packet of meat or fish doesn't have any labelling or explanation at all, don't even think about putting it in your basket because you are taking a risk with your health.

The problem with labels on food is that they aren't clear and they're misleading. Even some health foods are basically grains wrapped in sugar. A manufacturer will write 'plant-based' on the front, and that gives supermarkets permission to put it in the health-food section and whack the price up, when they're actually made from cheap, horrible ingredients.

'Plant-based' is the buzzword of the moment, but what plant are they made from? What industrialised crop that's depleting the earth of its ingredients is squeezed into that packet? Those plants are probably being grown in slurry and have so few nutrients.

I did a little experiment the last time I was in a supermarket. I picked up a couple of these jolly-looking plant-based snacks and had a look on the back of the packet. What a surprise to see our old friend sunflower oil was one of the main ingredients, as well as several different types of sugar.

After I had Jude, I wanted to lose some weight so I bought about thirty or forty commercially produced energy balls wholesale to save myself a bit of money from buying them individually. Before I knew it, I was eating ten a day and I couldn't stop.

I didn't allow myself to look at the ingredients on the back because I knew I would be horrified, so I waited until I was down to my last four and discovered they had four different types of sugars in them; all 'natural', all totally triggering. I might as well have been eating cookies (and they would have been much cheaper).

When you buy these foods, you're paying manufacturers to drive around in Range Rovers while they promote health and sustainability. That cereal you're buying because it had 'added vitamins' and cutesy packaging? It's likely to be made in the same factory as the supermarket's own brand. You're paying for the marketing, and for the big business owner's holidays to the Maldives.

You'll be surprised at how quickly you learn to read labels. It takes a bit of work initially, but before long it will become like second nature and you'll have a good, solid list of products you know you love and trust.

## FOOD SHOPPING

Food shopping can feel completely overwhelming when you're trying to be healthy. What's good for you? What's not? When you head to the supermarket my main advice would be to make the most of the first aisles (fruit and veg) and avoid the middle aisles (processed crap).

I try to spend the least amount of time possible in supermarkets because it's like being sucked into a void. I get in, get what I need and I don't deviate from my list. Once you start wandering down aisles you have no business being in, it's very easy to lose yourself.

We're set up to fail with the big supermarkets. As soon as you walk through the door, you're hit by the smell of freshly roasting chickens which are (not surprisingly) wafted around to make you feel hungry so you'll buy more.

The chances are, if you're nutritionally sound, those cravings won't kick in and you won't walk out with a tub of Rocky Road 'for the kids', and a multipack of Kit-Kats tucked under your arm so you can have a quick car snack. But if you're feeling wobbly, you could easily get sucked in.

Don't be that person who gets tricked by the big hitters. Have you ever been in to a health food shop that is pumping out the smell of tiger bread? No. Most of them smell of nuts and weird herbs, as they should do, because they're not trying to take advantage of your weak spots.

It goes without saying that you must never go to the supermarket feeling hungry. That's when they'll get you! Eat something solid and satisfying first. Don't go straight from a workout class or the gym feeling faint with hunger, because you will not come out with what you went in for, and your hungry body and mind will manage to find a way to justify why it's OK to buy giant bags of crisps.

Your nutrition devil and angel are fighting themselves more than ever in that moment, and how is the angel supposed to fight back if it's weak from a lack of nutrients?

When you're making decisions about what to buy, and you're being tempted by 'treats', ask yourself this question: 'Will I only eat one of those, or will I have to eat five? And will I still feel unsatisfied even if I do eat five? And will I have a terrible food hangover tomorrow?'

If you know you have no control when it comes to eating what you're buying, put it back on the shelf. If they're full of inflammatory oils, you'll be damaging yourself and your brain by having them, and you deserve better. And if you take your sugar and oil checklists with you, there is no excuse to buy the wrong things.

If you're really having a wrestle about whether or not you should have something, ask your gut. There's a reason people talk about 'gut feelings' or 'gut instinct' so much; because it's a real thing. Ask your gut if you should buy something and stick by its signals. I may sound a bit woo-woo here, but it works. Your body instinctively knows what is and isn't right for it.

## TIPS FOR EATING OUT

My first tip is to have a small protein shake before you go so you don't attack the bread basket because your blood-sugar levels are low and you're craving! I make a really simple shake out of a scoop of grass-fed whey protein powder and a banana whizzed up with some nut milk.

If you know you are going to be eating some inflammatory foods in a restaurant and it's unavoidable, then I recommend taking digestive enzymes before you eat to help your body process the junk (brands suggested at the back of the book). I feel these are worth investing in if you suffer from IBS or bloating, too. Digestive enzymes will help digest the food you eat, and you'll absorb the nutrition better, plus they also help with excretion.

I went for lunch with some friends and I took three digestive enzymes before, during and after the meal, and I didn't even have a hint of a food hangover. I felt a bit tired because I was digesting, but I wasn't in a food coma like I usually would be. I ate everything I wanted to, including tempura and white rice, but I was fine because I navigated my way around the 'bad' foods

– the tempura (I seemed to eat all of it) and the soy and sugars that were probably added to the food to make it taste so good.

You never see an ingredients list when you go to a restaurant, so I would assume if something tastes sweet and utterly delicious, it's because of what's been added to it!

Don't be afraid to ask restaurants what's in their food. Some places probably won't know because it's been shipped in ready-made, but if dishes are made from scratch, you can always ask them to leave something out or put something in.

Assume everything is factory farmed and not organic unless it is advertised as such.

Order the leanest cut of meat if it's not organic, because we know the toxins will be stored in the fat.

Ask for wild fish (you may be paying a ridiculous mark-up for farmed fish). Seabass is great, and ask for it to be fried in butter with herbs and seasoning, not oil.

Take your own stevia chocolate for dessert, and if you're going out to lunch and you know you'll want a coffee, take your own MCT powder to avoid a caffeine spike.

If you're not in the mood to stick to your programme, take notes on what triggered you to binge (were you tired or fed up?), and jot down how you feel afterwards. (Sleepy? Disappointed?) Write this down in your phone so you can refer to it afterwards. It might just help you to get back on track. Also take some activated charcoal tablets, which will bind to the inflammatory ingredients and mitigate as much damage as possible.

## MY 'SAFE' SHOPPING LIST

- **Soil Association**

- **Organic certification**

- **Outdoor bred**

- **Almond and cashew milk** have the best flavour, in my opinion.

- **Grass-fed butter** Grass is what cows are supposed to be fed on and will therefore contain more nutrients than butter from cows which are fed on grains and never go outside. Stay away from anything spreadable because it will contain inflammatory oils.

- **Raw milk and cream** from local farms because they have great nutritional values.

## INTERMITTENT FASTING

After six months of eating paleo, I started to experiment with intermittent fasting and as soon as I tried it, I knew it was going to work for me.

Intermittent fasting is when you increase the window in which you aren't eating, in order to allow your gut to rest. There are all sorts of different kinds of fasting regimes, from the 5:2 diet where you fast for two days a week, or the 18:6 diet where you eat for six hours a day and fast for eighteen. It's 'intermittent' because you're not fasting all the time. I mean, we need to eat.

Fasting isn't for everyone but it works well for me because I like to have boundaries. Sometimes if I start eating rubbish

I can't stop, so the best thing to do is not to start! I also need something to look forward to, and I get excited when I pick the kids up from school because I know we'll all eat together when we get home.

I used to be able to eat two whole pizzas, and then I'd go to the fridge to see what else was in there. Then I'd want dessert and then crisps. I didn't know how to moderate. But since I started fasting four years ago, I no longer get growling hunger pangs, and I'm not constantly looking around for something to put in my mouth.

I find that if I'm out and about it's really hard to find snacks or lunches that are healthy and in line with what I like to eat, and if I'm fasting that isn't an issue. I just wait till I'm home.

Your gut needs twelve hours to have a full clear-out between meals, and often people don't leave any time in between eating. They'll eat right up to bedtime, then wake up and have breakfast straight away. I like to think of fasting as a bit like when people are in an office for eight hours a day and then they go home and the cleaners come in. If they didn't allow the cleaners that time to work, the office would be disgusting, and it's the same with our bodies. They need a break to be able to clean themselves.

This process is called autophagy, which literally translates as 'self-eating'. What it means is that when we are in a fasted state, our body prioritises the removal of damaged cells, effectively cleaning up the body and restoring balance. You can think of it as like pressing a reset button back to optimal function. I totally get that this seems counterintuitive – we've been taught to eat little and often so that we don't get too hungry. But I've found the opposite is true; eating less often means I have fewer cravings.

You can train your body to get hungry at certain times. I've been told that the optimum intermittent fast is from 4 p.m. until 8 a.m. But I'm sociable and I want to be able to eat dinner with friends and my family, so I've fitted my fasting in around my family, because they're my priority. That means I fast for much of the day and eat with the family in the evening.

Fasting is totally normal in loads of different cultures, and I'm not sure when the whole snacking phenomenon kicked in. I don't snack because I don't go for the 'eat little and often' approach. Every time you eat you release insulin, and I believe you don't want constant spikes.

My parents wouldn't have snacked constantly when they were growing up because there wouldn't have been that much food around after the war. I'm sure snacking is a concept that was dreamed up by food companies, and studies have shown that it's healthier to give your body a break, rather than making it work to digest food all day long.

That's not to say I don't have mega slip-ups sometimes. When we first moved back up north in autumn 2020, I was eating cheese barm cakes (soft white rolls – eek!) like I'd gone on a Lancashire holiday. I ate fruit scones for the first time in thirty years, and things got so bad I was terrified I was going to veer into Pot Noodle territory.

I was stressed and feeling really ungrounded, and comfort food triggers oxytocin (which is also known as the 'cuddle' or 'love' hormone) and serotonin, which I needed at that time. It gives you an instant high and it distracts from the anxiety and the cortisol and uncomfortable emotions.

Even the process of buttering the bread conjured up old comforting memories, but I knew it was a simple case of self-sabotage. I went with it, tried my best to be kind to myself, and I was soon able to get back on the straight and narrow.

No one is perfect, and if we aim for perfection we will always fail because there is no such thing. I aim for 90/10, so I'm good for 90 per cent of the time, and I allow myself some leeway if I'm going out for dinner or doing something nice with the kids.

Intermittent fasting works for me because I know I'm not going to constantly spike my insulin by snacking. But I will have plenty of good fats, especially around my period when I'll be have cravings due to my hormones shifting and realigning.

Some women find it too tricky to fast for the second half of their hormonal cycle, when they are feeling particularly hungry, so don't bother if you don't want to. Your gut has already had a great rest for two weeks, so crack on with your breakfast if you need to.

If I have a fatty coffee with breakfast (see page 45 for recipe), I won't have carbs with it. I'll have something like scrambled eggs and smoked salmon and avocado, then I'll leave it a few hours before I tuck into some sourdough.

I love the fact that fasting means my gut is getting a proper chance to rest and digest all the food I've had the previous night. It can do its healing and go into autophagy, which is when the body recycles cells. All the dead calls get recycled and either chucked out or reused. You're giving your digestive system the time to do the clean-up.

Researchers believe autophagy is a survival mechanism that has anti-ageing benefits. As well as cleansing waste from the body, it provides energy, clears brain fog, reduces cravings and potentially fights cancer, neurodegenerative disease and other chronic illnesses.

One word of caution – however well it might work for you, don't start trying to put your kid on intermittent fasting. Children graze because they're growing, and they're moving a lot more than us. Well, not all of them, but I make sure my kids are doing something physically active every day. Intermittent fasting is fine after puberty, but not before. Children's guts are very easy to manipulate, which is a great and positive thing, but they need to be older before you start doing anything too extreme to their diets.

## How to start intermittent fasting

If you're new to intermittent fasting, start by doing twelve hours' fasting overnight. So you might finish eating by 8 p.m. and then have breakfast at 8 a.m., giving your gut a break to rest and digest.

At first I'd suggest you have three meals a day with at least a four-hour gap in between each meal. Make sure you have protein with each meal to keep you fuller for longer. Eggs are amazing for breakfast, or you could have a protein shake.

If you get shaky at times, it may mean you have imbalanced blood sugars, so you might need to snack on protein in between meals to keep you level. But you can train your body out of that over time. You might have previously trained it yourself by eating too much sugar and not enough protein and good fats at meal times.

Once your blood sugar has balanced out, you can start to extend the overnight fasting by an hour. You can even start by fasting twice a week and building up. You don't have to go hell for leather, which is something I would totally have done in the past.

When I first started fasting, it took me about a week to adapt into a twelve-hour fast, and then I extended it day by day until I eventually got to fifteen or sixteen hours. It took me about six weeks of really slowly building up to get to where I am now, where I don't eat a full meal until late in the day.

It amazes me that I can do it because I was that person who walked around supermarkets eating packets of biscuits and then had to send the empty packet down the checkout belt at the end. It definitely took some training to get out of my picking habits.

That's why you have to arm yourself before you go into the danger zones. If you're trying to stop yourself grabbing crap in the supermarket and you're only just starting out on the intermittent fasting journey, you need to make sure you're full of healthy fats so that you don't get tempted.

In the early days, I had to keep myself busy because I did get hungry at times. I also used to break my fast with celery juice because it's full of minerals and it would cleanse my tummy, and then I would start eating.

I often get asked if it's hard to exercise when you're fasting and I can honestly say that I find it really easy. In my experience it's possible to run about 15k in a fasted state, once you're used to it. Obviously take it easy at first – baby steps. But once you are fat-adapted, instead of running on glucose, you will find that you have so much energy. And of course you have to stay hydrated. I'm not always brilliant at remembering to drink water, but I do my best and drink when I'm thirsty.

## Make intermittent fasting work for you

I realise that my fasting schedule won't work for everyone, and it may take a bit of time for you to discover the best times for you to fast according to your daily schedule. I just worked out that I like to pick at night and that's how the time frame works best for me. If I want bacon and eggs for my dinner, I will have it. I don't really see meals in terms of categories now. I know it's traditionally a breakfast meal, but I love sitting down to that at 6 p.m.

I get so excited about night-time, when I'm able to have snacks and eat a cheeseboard on my bed with a litre of kombucha and *Succession* on telly. To me, that is heaven. Some people will want to eat breakfast and be happy to skip dinner instead. It's all about working out what works for you.

When I hear my tummy rumble these days, I know it's finished its recycling and I'm ready to eat. Normally if you hear your stomach rumble you've been going through mental torture trying to stop yourself eating, but these days I find that I don't get hungry until around 4 p.m. When I do, that's when I'll have carbs like sourdough or some sort of paleo bread, and a load of meat or eggs and avocados.

Whilst the kids are doing their homework or playing football, I'll have something nice to eat and then I'll start making dinner for all of us, which may be a beef stew or roast chicken and veg. If the kids want chips, I'll make them in an air fryer using organic potatoes and avocado oil. If we want a sweet treat, I'll make acai bowls, or we'll have some chocolate made with stevia instead of sugar. Stevia has no carbs, no calories and a glycaemic index of zero, meaning it doesn't raise blood sugar, so it's fine to have when you fast, too.

My staples for go-to meals are grass-fed beef, soups, eggs, avocados and salmon together, roast lamb, roast beef, and lots of shellfish with loads of garlic, the way the Spanish cook it. They're like comfort foods for me.

We do a lot of curries as well. Matthew makes them from scratch so they haven't got any nasties in them, especially if you use coconut oil and ghee (clarified butter), which is cheap, easily available and, according to Ayurveda, improves the absorption of the small intestine and is a rich source of omega-3 fatty acids, which decrease LDL cholesterol (often known as the 'bad' cholesterol because it increases your risk of health problems like heart attacks and strokes). We eat a lot of organic chicken thighs because they're much cheaper than breasts, and there's so much meat on them. I'm not sure who decided that breasts were best, but we've all been brainwashed into paying a fortune for something that isn't actually that tasty or as nutrient dense.

I also have at least one meal with shellfish in every week. Make sure you eat shellfish with a good fat like butter or olive oil, and a hit of vitamin C to help assimilate it more effectively. Put simply, you need vitamin C to absorb the benefits of fish, so even putting lemon on it is a good idea. I have mine with a small glug of fresh orange juice and a green salad on the side.

I always have a bowl of fruit out for the kids to graze on, but I don't really touch it until after 4 p.m. Some nutritionists are anti-fruit because of the sugar content, but I think that's taking things too far. Fruit is natural and in my opinion there's nothing wrong with eating it. Ancient man would have eaten fruit, and he would have eaten what was in season, which a lot of people advocate. It's easy enough to check online to see what's in season when, and the chances are those foods will be tastier and cheaper. This means having some stewed apples in the autumn rather than a mango smoothie. Or strawberries in the summer, when they're freshest and tastiest.

Eating seasonally is much better than eating trendily. I don't think we should be under pressure to eat what's on Instagram or being marketed that month. I didn't ever get into the whole kale thing. It's so spiky it even looks like it doesn't want to be eaten. I don't personally find it tasty either, and it makes me bloat.

The bottom line is, if you don't like the taste of something, don't eat it just because someone is telling you it's the key to a long life. You're not going to shorten your life just because you don't like blueberries and everyone bangs on about them being a superfood. To me, a true superfood is beef liver pâté because it will have a million times more nutrients in it than a blueberry smoothie.

One good tip is to have a protein-rich snack while you're making dinner. For me that is often either an egg, some bone broth with added fat and salt in it, or a protein shake – I aim for around 25g of protein per serving. This will satisfy you, meaning you won't be desperate for a dessert after you've eaten, or picking at the kids' leftovers.

People are sometimes scared of protein powders because they associate them with athletes or men trying to build big muscles in the gym, but protein isn't something to be feared, and unless you're on steroids you're never going to get arms like a body builder. Protein does build you up, but in a healthy, lean way.

I'll eat until 10 o'clock these days, and at some point in the evening I will watch Netflix with my feet up and enjoy a bowl of paleo cereal, which doesn't have agricultural grains in it. The one I have contains lovely things like nuts and coconut shavings and it's sweetened naturally with maple syrup or honey. I mainly have cashew milk or raw cow's milk, because I don't want the plant-milk stuff that is basically sugary water.

I take in more calories now, too. I eat thousands a day, but they're good ones which are nutritionally dense. I also try to eat a rainbow of foods, so as many different colours as possible because it's really good to have variety in your diet to keep your gut healthy.

I have at least one cup of bone broth a day to keep my gut strong. I can strengthen my stomach lining and support my mental and physical health (and protect myself from colds). It's a bit of a hazy area but I personally still think you get the benefits of fasting with a basic bone broth. If you add some fat to it, it will also fill you up. It may kick off the digestive system a bit, but it won't spike your insulin and it certainly won't be the same as having something like a bacon butty. It's a really good way to ease yourself into intermittent fasting. It's a change from coffee, it's really gut healthy and it's full of minerals. Bone broth is a good way to get you used to not snacking and grabbing a packet of something when you're peckish. It will make you feel satisfied without ruining all of your good work.

So there you have it. After much experimentation, I worked out that I prefer intermittent fasting and the paleo diet above everything. They suit my lifestyle and I have great energy and focus when I combine those two things.

A trick I've learned is that when I eat, I always stop and fast-forward twenty minutes and think about how I'm going to feel and weigh up whether it's worth it. Am I going to be satisfied? Am I going to bloat? And I going to be grumpy? If I answer yes to those last two questions, I'm not having it. I always think clean.

I don't see the way I eat these days as a 'diet' at all. It's my lifestyle now, and I feel better than I ever have. No one wants be lean but feel crap and miserable. What's the point in that?

It was my low self-esteem that used to panic me into fad diets, but when I lost a few pounds I would have a moment of elation, and then a huge comedown. That's probably because

I was nutritionally depleted from stupid food and my brain wasn't functioning well. If you deprive your body, you will send it haywire.

Nowadays, I don't need to diet because my muscles are constantly burning fat. I use food as a tool for my mental health, my gut health and my physical health. Food is medicine, and once you see it as that and you love the feeling of a sharp mind and a healthy body, you will begin to see food differently.

## Fatty coffee

One of the best tools in my intermittent-fasting arsenal is fatty coffee. I have found that this wakes me up and energises me for the day ahead, as well as helping to keep me full so that I don't crave sugary foods or carbs. I have it first thing, instead of breakfast, and throughout the day.

My fatty coffee (see recipe, page 45) is an adaptation of the famous 'bulletproof' coffee which was the brainchild of master biohacker and former Silicone Valley IT executive Dave Asprey. After ballooning to 21 stone due to a low-calorie, low-fat diet (yep!) and high cortisol levels from hardcore weightlifting, Asprey went on a journey of discovery to Tibet to learn to meditate and take better care of himself.

While he was trekking in the mountains, he was given a cup of tea infused with Yak's butter, which is said to give drinkers a clean caffeine high and promote weight loss. He was amazed at how alert he felt afterwards.

After returning to America, Asprey set about creating his own version, and eventually settled on a coffee, grass-fed butter and coconut oil combo which gives you a slower energy high, reduces jitters, kicks your body into fat-burning mode and keeps you fuller for longer. This helped him to lose 100 pounds. He then packaged and sold his formula and got very rich!

The irony is, I never used to be able to drink coffee without feeling really jittery and like I was coming down off something. I'd never been a coffee person. While everyone was going to coffee bars in the 90s off the back of watching *Friends*, I was very much still stuck in wine bars working my way through the mini fridges like I was in *Cheers*.

Then I listened to a podcast about the benefits of bulletproof coffee, and I decided to try it. I liked the calming feeling it gave me and the fact that the jitters had magically disappeared but I still had the energy from the caffeine.

MCT, aka medium-chain triglyceride, is a natural liquid oil that's derived from coconuts and doesn't get stored in the body. It's been shown to increase the release of peptide and leptin, which are two hormones that make us feel fuller, and therefore it helps to promote weight loss. It's also said to help reduce inflammation and candida.

I looked more into the science behind what Dave Asprey said and how the fat from the oil transports the caffeine through the brain and also takes away the jitters and the post-caffeine slump.

I was very overweight at the time I started making my fatty coffees, so I found the thought of having pure fat, in a coffee of all things, very scary. But I stuck to it, and I found that, when I drank it, I was less interested in snacks. Then I added stevia, which made it sweet and it tasted creamy. After a while I realised I found MCT oil a little bit heavy and I now prefer to use an MCT powder instead. But if I'm hungry and I don't have time to make a meal, or I'm trying to avoid that 11 a.m. snack, I'll whack some oil into a coffee and that will take the edge off my hunger.

I have a much better tolerance for caffeine now and I don't get the jitters, even with an espresso. But that is to do with the type of coffee you drink, too. Often coffee beans have mould and micro-toxins which cause anxiety, so go for the cleanest coffee you can. Always buy organic, and look out for the ones that state they are mould-free. If you can, get single-source coffee harvested from a high altitude. What you don't want is coffee that's been sitting around in a warehouse for days going mouldy before it's processed and packaged.

Fast-forward and I now use coffee as something that wakes me up in the morning, as a detoxifier and as a motivator.

Each morning, as soon as I get up, I'll have an espresso. I'll put a tablespoon of MCT oil or powder in there so it's like an emulsion. (Again, I find the powder is easier on my tummy than the oil.) You can also add butter, à la Dave. There are no hard and fast rules, but I find butter makes it a bit too heavy for me.

If the first thing you do in the morning is take in fat, that triggers your body into recognising fat and burning it as your fuel for the whole day, so you don't start craving sugars.

By having MCT oil I'm feeding my brain with good fats, and saving energy because (unlike digesting food) it doesn't tire you out. It's a different way to get energy, and intermittent fasting targets you into that zone where your body kicks in to use fat.

I've also become a fan of grating chaga mushroom into my coffee. It's a very powerful adaptogen, which is a herb or plant that helps to heal your body and relieve stress and anxiety. So it will help you to calm down during those moments when everything feels like it's going wrong! Chaga is also anti-inflammatory, relieves pain, stimulates your immune response, purifies the blood and protects the kidneys and liver. Oh, and it also helps with breathing, so it's great to have before I hit the gym or go for a run. What a genius all-rounder!

After a fatty coffee, I won't need to refuel until about an hour after I've worked out, at around midday. If you're doing high-intensity exercises, your body will try to use all of your carbs because they're easy to break down, but it will store your fat until all your carbs have gone, and then it will switch to breaking down fat. It's a lot more difficult for the body than burning carbs or sugar. With intermittent fasting and fatty coffee, you're training your body to use fat as fuel.

If coffee gives you the jitters, it may mean you have a certain type of genetic make-up which means you're not very good at metabolising caffeine, so I recommend using L-theanine supplements, which are said to inhibit the overstimulating effects of caffeine. I've gone from someone who found coffee too much to having several a day with no side effects. I think L-theanine is one of the best supplements out there. We're not talking fortunes here, either. Mine were around a tenner from Amazon.

If you're getting coffee while you're out and about, and you can't find a small organic coffee shop, I would recommend Pret A Manger over other coffee-shop chains because their coffee is organic. Add some powdered MCT oil and you're away.

When you're buying coffee for home use, make sure you use an organic mould-free coffee to get the brilliant benefits of the polyphenols (micronutrients), which are thought to help with weight management, digestive issues and diabetes (as long as you're not loading your coffee up with sugar).

Coffee is a brilliant antioxidant and it suits my diet and lifestyle, but I also have a break from it once a month so my body doesn't get too used it, or get intolerant. I'll use decaf instead for three to five days, before switching back to the hard stuff, but you'll find what works for you.

It may be that you want to do one week on and then a few days off. It all depends on how your body responds. My body is adapting and changing all the time, which means I am too, and now I'm in tune with it I can listen to what it needs.

A great alternative to coffee is matcha tea, which is powdered green tea and is great for autophagy (cell renewal, see above). It's also believed to be anti-inflammatory (another huge tick).

## DIETING AND DRINKS

People often forget about drinks when they're dieting. They'll clean up their diet, but they'll still drink loads of sugary or sugar-free 'diet' drinks. Just because something is liquid it doesn't mean it's OK to knock it back. It could contain all sorts of triggering ingredients.

If you stick to the 'count chemicals, not calories' mantra, it really makes you question things. You'll start looking at drinks that only have one calorie in them and thinking *Well, what is in them, then? They've taken out the sugar, but what have they added? And are those toxins going to sit in my liver and affect my brain? And are they going to spike my insulin and make me put on weight?*

**Green juices** Some people love green juices, and some people hate them. Some of them bloat me and make me feel crap, but there are other combinations that do work for me, which are mainly vegetable-based ones. There is so much sugar in some juices, it's unbelievable. If you take a ton of oranges and make a pint of freshly squeezed orange juice, it will have more sugar in it than a can of Coke.

Everyone's been going a bit mad about celery juice for the past few years because of a guy called The Medical Medium. He became really big on Instagram thanks to the Kardashians, but he's a bit woo-woo for me. I was still interested in trying the juice, which is so simple as all it involves is you drinking the juice of a bunch of celery on an empty stomach first thing in the morning. We're not talking rocket science here.

My take on the whole celery-juice phenomenon is that it's not going to cure every illness in the world, but it's great rehydration, it provides lots of electrolytes, minerals and vitamins and it's a brilliant laxative. The water is really available in that it gets into your cells well, and it's pretty cheap.

If you find it hard to stomach, you can mix it with cucumber to dilute the 'interesting' taste. I have celery juice twice a week when I break my fast, and I definitely feel the effects (if you get my drift).

**Drink swaps** Matthew loves Diet Coke (sigh), but he also likes Gallybird tonic water, which is much better for you as it's sweetened with stevia. So I stock up on that to try and lure him away from the aspartame.

Even though Diet Coke is sugar free, it's got sugar-mimicking ingredients, so it will still spike your insulin and hamper weight loss. People will always drink Diet Coke, so I'm hoping it's just a matter of time before someone brings out an organic Coke with stevia in it.

**Energy drinks** I steer clear of energy drinks because many contain some truly awful ingredients, and often a ton of caffeine and sugar. Have a coffee instead! If you do want to have an energy drink, take L-theanine with it to counteract the caffeine jitters. Also have some chlorella, which is a super-absorbent algae that binds on to the toxins and preservatives that give energy drinks a long shelf life.

**Chia gel drink** Another good way to get hydration into yourself is to mix chia seeds into water so they form a gel. Your body absorbs gel much better than water, so you'll feel hydrated for longer. This is great if you're in a hot environment or working out.

I crush my chia seeds up using a pestle and mortar to increase the surface area. Add some nice purified water and then wait for it to turn to gel, which takes a few hours, or just leave it overnight in the fridge. It morphs into H3O2, meaning it has an extra hydrogen and oxygen atom, therefore it increases the surface area, and our cells absorb it better. You'll be getting your recommended two litres of water by having only one litre of water, and you won't wee out the minerals. You also won't need to get up to wee in the night, which is always a bonus. It's how a lot of long-distance runners keep themselves hydrated.

**Water filter** I make sure my water is as pure as it can be, but I don't want to pollute the world by buying bottles of purified water in single-use plastic bottles. Instead, I've got a filter to remove all the nasties, like chlorine, bacteria, lead and parasites, which can all be detrimental to our health in different ways.

My filter has huge cylinders filled with activated charcoal. It's very simple because as the water drips through, it sucks all the chlorine out. The activated charcoal is highly absorbent, so it binds to toxins like chlorine and removes them.

I'll add lemon and a pinch of salt to the kids' water to put some minerals back in, as the charcoal takes those out too.

I know it costs money to buy water filters, but up to 60 per cent of the human body is water, and we need to feed those cells the best way we can. This kind of water is easier for our cells to absorb.

Matthew, the kids and even my dogs drink the filtered water, and when I think about the money I save on buying bottled water, it's worth it in the long term.

**Protein shakes** I have a love/hate relationship with protein powders. They're so convenient, particularly if your period is due and you need to increase your protein levels to avoid cravings. However, a lot of non-organic, vegan powders and mass-produced powders are so full of sugar and crap, you might as well eat a Mars bar. Also, stay away from soy-based powers, because soy is highly processed.

I found an amazing protein powder that uses organic whey protein (see page 242 for recommended suppliers). Another one I've found has got four different types of protein from organic grass-fed beef, chicken, fish and egg shells, all in one unflavoured protein.

If I can't be bothered to make a meal and I'm hungry, I'll add some cashew milk and a banana to the protein powder so it's really palatable.

If you're vegan or dairy intolerant, go for pea protein, which is a source of protein extracted from green and yellow split peas.

**Olive oil** OK, so I know olive oil isn't strictly a drink, but I *do* drink it. I had no idea how powerful it was until I read up on it, but it's incredible stuff. It protects against inflammation, it contains loads of antioxidants, it may help prevent strokes and it protects against heart disease. It also has anti-bacterial properties, meaning it can kill or inhibit harmful bacteria we have in our bodies.

Extra virgin olive oil is the least processed form of olive oil, so it retains its natural antioxidants and vitamins, which can be lost during processing. It means it's more expensive than other olive oils, but it's much healthier.

I have two tablespoons of a high-quality organic olive oil every time the pain in my right hip flares up. You need to have a water and lemon chaser because it doesn't taste great, but I have found it definitely helps with aches and pains.

## COOKING AND KIDS

I would never in a million years feed my kids according to the NHS guidelines. The current recommendation is that a third of your diet should be made up of whole-wheat pasta, cereals and breads. Another third should be fruit and vegetables, and then they've lumped lentils and meat in the same category because they're both proteins. Oh, and they recommend spreads instead of butters. WTF?!

Everything on the latest advice list seems to spike your insulin, because they're taking pointers from doctors who were taught about nutrition twenty years ago.

The health landscape has changed so much, so why are we still listening to such old-fashioned advice? Throw in the fact that most of the government guidelines are funded by the sugar and agricultural industries and you've (literally) got a recipe for disaster.

When I followed these guidelines, I put on weight, I had low energy, I couldn't get out of bed because I was so tired, I experienced monumental cravings and I was extremely bloated. Apart from that, it was great!

The government saying things like 'we need moderation' doesn't help anyone. Especially when you have advertising subliminally pushed through your TV on a daily basis. Why are we not being given genuinely decent advice?

My friend's mum was referred to an NHS nutritionist because she had gallbladder and stomach issues and was told she needed to follow quite a specific diet.

She was sitting in the waiting room at the hospital before her appointment when this really large woman came out of a room and called her name. My mate's mum couldn't stop herself from thinking, *My God*, that *woman needs to go and see a nutritionist*. But yep, you guessed it, that woman *was* the nutritionist.

She also gave her all sorts of bad advice, like eating really low-fat foods, that my friend's mum knew wasn't right because she's read a lot of books and done a lot of research herself. What a waste of money for the NHS!

I would say always try to cook from scratch and the fewer ingredients you use during cooking, the better. Unless you're using natural ingredients to flavour your food, like a clove of garlic, an onion and some rosemary.

Don't go for the packaged herbs and spices if you can help it. Why do you need to buy a tube of pre-prepared garlic with additives when the real thing is cheaper, natural and tastes so much better? I totally get that it's about convenience (I'm someone with four kids), but that extra minute it takes to chop up a few cloves of garlic makes all the difference.

I will add salt to food and I don't know why it's been demonised. So many people are low in essential minerals found in sea salt. The best place to find it is in good-quality sea salt like Maldon, rather than the cheap processed stuff.

Children like sweet things because they're high energy and

they themselves are growing. As adults, we don't need as many sweet things because we're not growing. If you like vegetables, great, ferment them and prepare them so your kids will like them more. My kids love roasted veg with pesto, or I'll cut raw veg into strips and serve them with hummus or avocado mayo.

Parents have been told they have got to make kids eat more greens. We're taught to give them spinach, like Popeye, but you'll get more iron in a steak. I slice it up for the kids and I add a garlic mayonnaise which is mainly made from avocado oil.

My kids need more nutrition than me as they are growing brain cells and muscle mass, so I make sure they have the best-quality food I can find. I do not want them to go through what I went through in the 80s and 90s, being addicted to processed food that caused depression and weight gain.

I'm not a big milk user, but I'm going to start reintroducing milk to the kids' diet a bit more. It's a source of good bacteria and amazing building blocks that the gut needs to function well. A lot of people vilify dairy and think it's really bad for you, but I personally have never had an issue with it. I don't think it's healthy to cut out entire food groups from your diet unless you have an allergy or a genuinely strong reaction to them.

I get that some people avoid eating healthily because they think it's confusing or expensive, and they've got families to think about. But you honestly can feed your family like your feed yourself. Just make tweaks.

One lady messaged me saying that she and her husband decided to change the way they ate long term. They shelved the processed foods and made their dinners from scratch every night. They cut out gluten and sugar as much as possible and also started off doing light exercises, before building up to running.

Within four months they had both lost loads of weight and were feeling so much better. They both had loads more energy too, so they were doing more activities with their two teenage kids, like long walks and bike rides. However, what they noticed was that their kids got tired easily and all of a sudden they were the fit ones. The reason for that? While they were cooking themselves these amazing dinners, the kids were coming home from school and eating meals like fish fingers, chips and beans for their tea, which is basically a bunch of empty calories. They were still eating like they always had, so they weren't benefiting from all the extra fruit and veg like their parents were.

After a bit of bribery, the kids agreed to do an experiment and eat the same food as their parents for a month, and it doesn't take a genius to guess what happened. They got leaner, their mood lifted, they needed less sleep and they didn't struggle to get up for school each morning. They felt sharper in class and more motivated to exercise.

While I do understand it can be tricky to get your whole family involved in your new way of eating, it can be done, especially if you lead by example.

If you've got little ones, start them young. My boys will happily have green juices, but I make theirs a bit sweeter than I make my own. You can't expect a six-year-old to willingly drink liquid kale and cucumber.

I try my best to keep rubbish food out of the house and the kids do eat really well, but of course sometimes they want to have the same things as their mates at school. It would be unfair if they didn't. I never called sweets 'treats'. A treat is some new football boots or a bath bomb from Lush, which they love. I also get organic bovine gelatine, which is really good for making sweets using real juice.

# Homemade jelly sweets

These contain just two ingredients. It's worth looking at the ingredients on a packet of jelly sweets by way of comparison – this has got to be better for your kids!

250ml pure fruit juice
2 tbsp organic bovine gelatine

- Add the fruit juice to a pan and warm it up, but don't let it boil. Stir in the gelatine until it's fully dissolved.

- Pour the mixture into sweet moulds, which you can pick up from any kitchen shop.

- Stick them in the fridge for one to two hours until they're set, and then pop them out of the moulds.

- Ta-da! Instant sweets.

~

My kids do have sugar on Hallowe'en and their birthdays because I'm not evil, but I do try and keep it to a minimum. If they go to a kids' party, they'll have a load of junk but they notice how they feel afterwards and they hate it. They'll get really high, then really tired, and then really cross with me, even though I didn't give them the sweets. Acer will say, 'I don't like it, I feel sick.'

It doesn't give me pleasure giving them crap. It's like a positive affirmation telling them that sugar is a treat. Do that with alcohol when you get older, and look what happens to some of us. I'm an addict and they're 50 per cent my kids, so I'm going to err on the side of caution.

I've always got fruit bowls around and they will naturally gravitate towards fruit because they really like it. I try to make what they eat functional for them so there's a reason for it to be there and they're not just mindlessly eating.

I think when the kids get to about thirteen or fourteen their gut microbiome will be established, and hopefully I'll have set them on the right trajectory. I really want them to be well and happy and healthy, and I believe this gives them the best foundation.

## A FEW SHOCKING FOOD HOME TRUTHS TO END ON

- You would think that something that is sold as cream was cream, right? Read the back of some of the popular brands and you'll be very surprised. One 'cream' in particular is actually made up of E numbers, powders, soya, veg oils and colourings. There is no actual cream to be found.

- White basmati rice is better for you than brown rice. I know, it's shocking, but brown rice contains anti-nutrients, which stop you getting the minerals from food by blocking absorption. And, if you ask me, white basmati tastes nicer too. Pippa Campbell was telling me that the nutritional world has done a turnaround on brown rice and they don't recommend it any more. Who could have seen that coming?

- When you think about fibre, you generally think about breakfast cereals that taste like a bit of old door mat, or baked beans, both of which bloat you up and give you chronic wind. In my opinion, that kind of fibre has been invented to make us think our bodies won't function without it, when in fact fibre is in everything from meat to vegetables and nuts. You see it all the time on food packaging which boasts that it's a 'great fibre provider'. We don't need to spike our insulin and get fat just so we can hit our fibre target. If you get a chance, look up the sugar content of 'healthy' breakfast cereals. You will be horrified.

## SO HOW'S YOUR FOOD?

I hope I've given you some things to think about when it comes to the food you eat, and the food you feed to your loved ones. I know there's a lot to take in, and I get that there's so much confusion between the official NHS guidelines and what I'm suggesting. That's where you need to become your own expert. Don't take my word for it.

Use your mood and food journal and start noticing how you feel if you remove inflammatory foods from your diet. Try a fatty coffee for breakfast one day and see if intermittent fasting is for you.

There's always going to be some new superfood, or another fad diet that promises to change your life. But I promise you that when you eat real food, as close to Mother Nature as possible, and in line with your body's needs, you won't ever need another diet again.

## DAVINIA'S TOP FIVE FOOD TAKEAWAYS

- Eat food as close to its natural state as possible
- Stop counting calories, start counting (and avoiding) chemicals
- Read labels to avoid hidden sugars and vegetable oils where you'd least expect them
- Add good fats to your diet, ditch all low-fat and 'diet' foods
- Give your gut a break with intermittent fasting.

# MOVEMENT

I would love to say that my health journey was seamless and that as soon as I started eating more healthily, I hit the gym and took up running. But *no.*

Even though I knew that eating well and exercising should go hand in hand, at the beginning I felt too fat and embarrassed to go to a gym. I thought everyone was going to be a size zero and dressed head to toe in Lululemon. I had never been one to exercise, other than dancing in nightclubs, so it felt really alien to me. It wasn't like I'd been really into fitness at any point and then fallen off the wagon, I hadn't ever been *on* the wagon to start with, and the only lycra I owned was left over from my clubbing days (it was acceptable back then, honest).

But as I'm going to explain, just because you've never been into fitness doesn't mean you can't find your pathway into it. I may have taken a bit of a wriggly route to fitness, but once I got the benefit of exercise, I *really* got it, and it has changed my life for the better. Not just on a physical level – although it is a blessing that my bum cheeks no longer feel like they're banging on the back of my knees – but on a mental-health one too.

I could not live without exercise now. It wasn't until I started feeling better that I realised how shit I'd felt before. I thought I was 'normal' back then, but my God, I could not go back to feeling like that now. Not for anything.

What I've learned over the years is that being healthy may feel like hard work at first, but being unhealthy is even harder.

## I HAVE NEVER BEEN A NATURAL EXERCISER

I wasn't that person that came out of the womb wearing a pair of running shoes, and I didn't do dance or karate lessons for fun like some of my mates did when we were kids.

I was OK at sport at school, but I didn't particularly enjoy it. I was never the fastest, and I've got this deep competitive dopamine-type personality that has to win. I've got an all-or-nothing mentality, so if I didn't come first, I didn't see the point.

My dad was hugely competitive at school and was a champion hurdler for the Liverpool Schoolboys, so I feel like I get that drive from him. My mum was useless at any sort of sport. I had my dad's will to win, combined with my mum's 'talent'. So basically, it was a nightmare.

I didn't mind team sports, so I joined in with those, but only because they were on the timetable. The idea of exercising for enjoyment or using exercise as a mental-health strategy was completely alien to me. Like most people, I had no idea about the uplifting benefits of exercise or how good it is for building self-esteem.

I was at a sporty school, so we were expected to get our gym shorts on and get out there, and every time we had to do cross country, obviously I would feign sickness or say I had terrible period pains. The one time I did do the run I came fourth out of everyone, which I was really surprised about. But it was just so fucking awful and took so long, I decided I would never do it again. I later found out in my genetic test that I do have a genetic predisposition to do long distance, so I'm good at being slow and steady.

Even after I left school, there was no point where I started to enjoy exercise. I got straight into drinking and partying. There was zero exercise whatsoever. There was nothing except staying up all night. That was my endurance.

There was no gym membership. No swimming. Nothing. All I would do was go on a crash diet before I went on holiday with a supermodel (and it never worked either: I always hid my body in kaftans instead).

Back in my late teens and early twenties, I was so tired I couldn't even imagine going to a gym anyway. There were a few times when I tried whatever exercise class was trending. I tried Zumba and I was terrible. I've got no coordination and I hated it. I tried kickboxing and again, hated it. I know people who love it, but I always thought to myself *I'd be having a much better time in the pub*.

I thought the gym was for losers, but I think that's because I was a bit jealous that other people could do it and seemed to like it. I didn't have the energy, and I didn't have the inclination. If I did dip my toe in, I didn't get a buzz from it, it just hurt. I didn't realise exercise could actually help with my mood if I persevered. I thought I had to take a prescription pill for that.

My problem was that none of my mates were really exercising either. Back then, it was the height of ladette culture and it was all about drinking and partying. I think girls who are in their twenties now have far better influences, particularly because you don't have to look a certain size, and it's all about wellness, whereas back then it was about staying up all night and how many pints you could drink, and whether you could match the blokes.

After I got sober, I decided to try and exercise. But I couldn't exercise my way out of the inflammation because of my crazy diet and the effect my fake boobs were having on my body. I had the headspace and the time to try different kinds of exercise, but because I was still feeling big, I didn't run.

I also had three more pregnancies in my thirties, and I was on a lot of anti-depressants as well, so I felt very flatlined throughout. It was a case of me having to drag myself into the gym to try and make myself feel better. But because I was on bipolar medication, I didn't get the uplifting buzz from working out that I do now. I wasn't getting those amazing highs that make pushing yourself worth it.

I don't feel like I wasted that time in my thirties, because I was experimenting. It takes a lot of trial and error before you find something you like. I mean, I know yoga is shit for me. I hate it. I tried it for years. I tried to be one of the trendy set and be all 'ohhmmm', but it doesn't work for me. I don't get a buzz from it.

People tell me how free and amazing the yoga moves make them feel and tell me not liking it is a problem with my mind, and maybe it is, because it makes me feel claustrophobic. But at least I gave it a go. I tried Bikram, transcendental yoga, meditation – you name it, I've done the courses.

If you had told my twenty-seven-year-old self that I'd be running marathons in my forties, I would have rolled my eyes and thought *as if!* My imagined future had me chainsmoking all day and drinking champagne.

What you discover when you get sober is that things don't all magically fall into place. They get a million times better, but you still have to put in the effort to change other things in your life that aren't working. So it took me a while for that effort to pay off.

As someone who is dopamine driven and serotonin depleted, I need more than sobriety. I need a buzz. I just had no idea I would end up getting that from running.

## GET KITTED OUT

When I first began thinking about embracing exercise, I thought if I bought some really amazing workout clothes they would make me want to work out. I know that really helps some people (if it helps you, get those Sweaty Betty leggings immediately!). But I soon realised it wasn't about having the fanciest leggings or sports bra. At that point, nothing would have made me go to the gym.

In the end, I forced myself to go to H&M and stock up, because their range is really good, reasonably priced and they do bigger sizes. I thought that at least if I didn't make it to a class, I wouldn't have wasted loads of money.

I started wearing my fitness gear around the house just to get used to myself wearing exercise clothes. I genuinely think that helped me get into a better mindset about it all. Spanx do their own workout gear now and if I'd known back then I would definitely have got some of that as well. I would really have welcomed the extra help in the beginning to feel like I was ready to exercise.

I massively suggest that you either dig out your old exercise gear or invest in some new stuff. Like I said, it doesn't have to be expensive. But psychologically, when you put on fitness clothes, you are telling yourself that you're someone who exercises. And that is half the battle, I promise.

Back then, I was always making excuses for myself, and I'd be the first to tell people I'd had four children to try and excuse how big I was. I still felt too big to run, but I started to feel more comfortable in fitted clothes, so I started going out and about in them. I wore three-quarter-length black leggings on the school run and to the supermarket and they became like a second skin.

Within two weeks of changing my eating patterns and wearing workout gear, I had a shift. It was like a part of my brain was saying to me 'Look, you've got the clothes now, so you may as well start *actually* exercising'.

Even though I hadn't lost tons of weight by then, mentally I felt like I'd moved forward and my inflammation was calming down, so I liked what I saw in the mirror a bit more. I don't think other people would have been able to notice a difference in me, and I didn't drop much on the scales, but I felt less bloated and inflamed and I noticed that my water retention had gone down.

My belly looked flatter, which was a massive thing for me. I know it sounds naff but it gave me a bit more of a spring in my step, and made me want to feel even better. When your tummy sticks out, clothes don't seem to hang on you as well, and I always felt so self-conscious about my stomach. Even if I put on a baggy T-shirt, I felt like it clung to me.

I also think once you rid your brain of inflammation you feel lighter, and the knock-on effect was that I started having healthier thoughts about myself.

As a general rule, I'm not a big one for weighing myself. I am 5'5" and I weigh between eight and a half and nine stone, fluctuating depending on where I am in my cycle or the time of year. I tend to eat more lightly during the summer months.

I think it can be dangerous to weigh yourself too often because it can become a decider as to whether you feel happy or sad, or you have a good or bad day.

I really suggest that you focus on how you *feel*, rather than what you weigh. This is always the best guide, rather than a fluctuating number on a scale.

I was so embarrassed the first time I went back into a gym after so long away. But do you know what I soon realised? You don't have to own the coolest exercise gear in order to be let through the door of a gym.

No one else actually gives a shit about how you look. The chances are they were once bigger too; they've just been working out and eating well for longer. No one is born with amazing muscle definition and a high tolerance for cardio. We all get there from somewhere.

I promise you that if someone is going to a gym in a bid to look better, they're going to be concentrating on their own progress, not whether the woman on the next treadmill is carrying a few extra pounds.

Here's a home truth for you. That size-eight woman in the leggings and matching crop top in the front row of your class isn't looking in the mirror so she can see if you're doing all the exercises the correct way or not. She's too busy thinking about the next bit of the class, and how hard she's worked to look that good. And quite right too!

## WALKING BACK TO HAPPINESS

The first thing I did in the gym was get on a treadmill. I walked on an incline and set a pace of 3km an hour to test myself out and see how fit/unfit I was. I put on my earphones and played some disco music, and that made me feel happier and more motivated. I speeded things up a bit, and when I got a proper sweat on after thirty minutes, I felt like I was doing something right.

Before I started biohacking, I always assumed that to burn fat you had to really *feel* the burn, and push yourself incredibly hard. It surprised me to learn that pushing your heart rate too high takes you *out* of fat-burning mode.

You never see a bodybuilder run before they do a show, because that will put them into a cardio burning workout. That means they've got past the fat-burning zone and into a heart-training zone. Cardio is great for fitness if you want to increase your heart rate to do something like mountain running. But if a bodybuilder wants to cut fat and show off their muscles, they will walk on an incline for hours so they stay in the fat-burning zone and lose weight.

People often think that harder is better, but if you want to drop weight quickly you need to bring the effort down, so your body doesn't think you're in survival mode and start storing energy. When you push yourself too hard, your body goes into stress mode and your cortisol immediately increases, which can lead to sleep issues, digestive problems and weight gain.

So if your goal is to burn fat, I reckon it's worth investing in a heart-rate monitor (I use the one on my Apple watch) so you can keep track of your BPM or heartbeats per minute.

## Your optimal fat-burning zone

Here's how to work out the BPM you need to aim for in order to burn the most fat.

Subtract your age from 220. This gives you your *maximum* BPM, which is well above the fat-burning zone.

Then multiply that number by 0.7 to give you 70 per cent. That is your BPM limit for fat burning – any time your heart rate goes above that number, you are into the cardio zone and out of fat burning.

So if you are thirty-five years old, you would take 35 away from 220, which equals 185. That would be your maximum BPM. Your ideal fat burning zone needs to be 70 per cent of that, which would be 130.

Mine works out at 123, so my heart rate shouldn't go above 123 beats per minute because otherwise I'll go into cardio, which means I'm then exercising my heart, and I want fat loss.

I go slowly and steadily and I check my BPM on my Apple Watch or via my Oura Ring/iPhone as I'm walking to make sure I don't go above 123 BPM. When I'm in that mode I'm a bit out of breath but I can still hold a conversation.

## My favourite fat burner

If I've got a decent chunk of time, my favourite fat-burning exercise is the 6/6/60 treadmill power walk.

I do a 6 per cent incline at 6km per hour for 60 minutes.

Then I do a 3 per cent incline at 3km per hour for (you guessed it) 30 minutes.

Try it for yourself. You'll sweat, you'll improve your mood and you'll burn fat more effectively than you would in a HIIT class.

Don't worry if the incline feels too hard at first, just bring it down a bit. Even a 1 per cent incline is going to work your glutes, which are the biggest muscles in your body. If you're working your glutes, you're instantly burning calories.

## BUT I HATE EXERCISING!

Look, we all have those days where we wake up and we just can't be arsed. It's cold, it's wet, or maybe you're just not in the mood. Before you give yourself a hard time about it, it's worth realising it's not laziness, it's just your brain doing what it's been designed to do over millions of years, which is self-preservation.

Your primal brain has learned to conserve energy at all costs in case you need to run away from danger, or there's no food to be found, so it's telling you to rest and save your energy for when you really need it. The only thing you can do is override it – overrule your primal brain and break through that pain barrier of getting moving. After a few minutes your brain and body will respond and you'll be on a roll. You'll be rewarded with some endorphins and you'll soon be feeling bloody great and you'll have a great day.

There's nothing worse than thinking you should be doing something and not doing it. Actually doing it is better than the mental torture that we go through trying to make excuses for ourselves. Don't let your primal brain get in the way of your body's capabilities and the life you want for yourself.

Exercise is like a hangover before the party. It may feel like the last thing you want to do, but you're going to get that amazing high afterwards, which will make it all worth it.

I've had quite a few people contact me online to see if I can help them with their weight problems or their bloating. I am happy to help anyone, but with the best will in the world, I knew a couple of them were reaching out to me for a magic bullet, and they really didn't want to hear that they might need to exercise three or four times a week.

I totally get that exercising feels daunting, and often you'd rather sit on the sofa instead. But if you do what you've always done, you're not going to change anything. If you're leaving your weight loss and fitness up to other people, it's never going to happen. If you don't work out, you won't get the highs or that feeling of achievement. Nobody can do that for you, or feel those feelings for you.

Although I found starting was hard, working out became very rewarding very quickly because I started to have more energy in my everyday life. I got hooked on that feeling of being able to get out of bed without moaning about it for half an hour, and noticed that I was ever so slightly less angry if someone cut me up in the car. Not only was I feeling better because I looked better, I noticed that my stress levels went down because I was burning that excess anxiety off by exercising.

I was able to make proper plans and know I would be able to stick to them. I'd had times where I'd been so tired I'd had to cancel things, but now I felt more confident that when Saturday night rolled around I wouldn't be in an energy deficit and I would be fine to meet friends for dinner.

I was putting out more energy by working out, but I discovered that I was getting more energy back, which I found shocking. It really made me question all the times I'd made the excuse that I was too tired to work out. In actual fact, some of the times I went for a run feeling groggy and exhausted were some of the times I felt best afterwards, like I'd shaken that tired feeling off.

But I also had times where I felt completely exhausted after hardly doing anything. I always say give your body at least two full weeks to get back into an exercise regime.

I don't have a fixed amount that I exercise each day or week. These days, I am so in tune with my body that I know when I do and don't need to work out. If I feel a bit sluggish, I won't use that as an excuse not to exercise, because sometimes the very thing I need is to get out in the fresh air and feel a bit of nature around me. I'm not into tree-hugging or anything, but the visual stimulation seems to help with my brain function and energy, even if I'm just having a walk.

If it's winter and the cold weather has kicked in, I have to make sure I have everything I need to make my outside exercise session a success. I need gloves, because I get cold hands; I need a Flipbelt, because I can't run with my phone in my hands; my headphones have to be fully charged so that I can listen to house music and pretend I'm nineteen again.

Work out what your excuses are and find a way to get past them. The only person you're cheating by avoiding exercise is yourself.

## KEEP ON RUNNING

Once I'd got the hang of the gym treadmill, I decided to really ramp things up and start walking/running each morning. It was agonising going out in the cold and dark, and I walked more than I ran in the beginning, but music and audiobooks got me through.

After a few weeks of walking every weekday (with a little bit of jogging thrown in) I began to notice more fat loss, particularly around my waist. I thought I was stuck with loose skin and love handles after four pregnancies. Until then I'd been doing full-on HIIT classes but my body was still holding on to excess fat, and I couldn't understand why.

When I looked into it, I discovered that my body was storing the belly fat in case of emergency because I'd been doing a lot of stress-inducing exercise. I thought I was doing the right thing hitting the cardio hard, but my poor body was panicking that I was in danger.

When the body is stressed, it releases more cortisol which is the 'fight-or-flight' hormone that responds to a perceived danger. When cortisol levels stay high – because of constant stress, and also stress-inducing exercise – the body will seek out sweet and fatty foods as it may need fast-acting energy. Comfort eating, anyone? And, worse, cortisol causes the body to hold on to excess weight, especially around the middle of the body.

It's counterintuitive, I know, but slowing down your exercise routine may actually be the best way to get lean for good.

By walking and breathing more steadily, I'd calmed my system down and levelled out my cortisol levels so my body felt safer and began to release its grip on my belly overhang. Now I realise the importance of getting the right balance between high-intensity workouts and allowing my body to rest and relax.

I read a great book called *Born to Run*, which explained that you're going to burn more fat running 5k in forty minutes than you would if you did it in thirty minutes. Pushing yourself out of the fat-burning zone and into the cardio zone doesn't help you lose weight, so pull it back and slow down.

Running is one of the most natural things a human can do. In evolutionary terms, we have only stopped doing longer-distance walking and running really recently.

Believe it or not, we're built to run long distance better than dogs. They have to stop and pant, but we can keep going because we have two to four million sweat glands all over our body so we can keep ourselves cool as we run. Dogs rely on panting to cool them down or they will overheat. That's how we used to be able to run down our prey when we evolved as hunter gatherers.

It's totally fine to stop and start when you're running. Go at your own pace to start with. There is no shiny first-place cup waiting for you at the end. It's just you and your heartbeat and your lungs and your brain.

I like to think of a run as a big washing machine doing a really deep, thorough wash of your body every time you go out there. You're breathing deeper, you're getting more oxygen to your brain and your body. It's like a form of meditation.

The whole point of fat burning is to exercise for as *long* as you can, not as *hard* as you can. Don't wear yourself out straight away so you can only last two minutes. Pace yourself. If I'm on the treadmill I'll still step off to get my breath back every now and again.

I took to running and jogging much more easily than I expected, and I reckon if I'd lived back in cavemen times, I would have been that person who was constantly running between all the different tribes so I could spread news and gossip. And I love to get the pay-off from the endorphin rush (once an addict . . .). Endorphins are the hormones your pituitary gland produces to decrease anxiety, block pain and create feelings of euphoric happiness. Endorphins are chemically similar to morphine. So let's face it, it's no wonder we like them so much.

I never thought I would say this, but sometimes now I run

5k, or 10k or even 15k a day. I was the woman who only liked to get out of bed for a party and had to start off walking because running was too hard. Now it's like second nature to me.

If you have any kind of back or knee problems and you can't run, walking on an incline is amazing and will give you similar results. You'll actually probably burn more fat than you would by running. If you walk every day with an incline, you are going to lean up so fast.

All movement starts in your mind, so get your head fired up with some tunes you love. Music is such an essential for me. I am not mentally strong enough to sit with silence for an hour's workout. I think I would go mad.

Build up your stamina: run for the chorus and walk for the verse. You don't even have to do all of the choruses: start with one. You'll soon start building up strength and music makes the time whizz by. Sometimes the banging tunes are the only thing that will get me out of the door and into a park, class or gym.

## PERFECTION IS A MYTH

Don't aim for perfection because you can only fail. We're never going to be perfect, because we compete with ourselves on a daily basis, and some days you feel great and ready to do a great run, and others you may feel horribly hormonal and want to hide away from the world.

We have to accept those fluctuations in our physical strength and our moods and know that every day can't be amazing, but if we keep going we're going to have a lot more good days than bad. It's all about feeling as good as we possibly can, and knowing that if we have a down day, if we take the right supplements, eat well and do a bit of exercise – no matter how light – the next day will be better.

If you push yourself too much during times of stress, guess what? You're going to stress your body out even more and you could end up getting ill. If I'm having a rough day there's no way I'm going to go to Barry's Bootcamp to half-kill myself. I'll go for a leisurely jog to keep my mental health in check, but I won't give myself a hard time because that will be really detrimental to my mood.

If you really can't cope with exercise, a cold shower is a smart way to get some endorphins (see page 181). And then give yourself a break.

If you want to move but make it relaxing, put on some good music and go for a speedy walk. It's load-bearing on your legs and I think we're all built to walk. Set yourself a goal of doing 7,000 steps a day and build up from there.

As we get older, resistance training is really good, especially around the perimenopause and menopause, when our muscle mass decreases and fat mass increases (argh!). Working out with some resistance bands will help you to build up muscle, and it can easily be done at home. I would also recommend doing weights. Even doing five reps will activate your muscles.

Whatever you choose to do, it has to be sustainable. What's the point in doing something for a month and then finding yourself going back to your old habits six months down the line because you've set unrealistic goals?

If you can't exercise because you're not well or you've got an injury, you've got to be careful that your mood doesn't dip and you end up reaching for the biscuit tin. If I'm really not in the mood to exercise, or nursing an injury, I will still go for walks, more for my mental health than anything.

I had a whole week of not being able to exercise when I was going through some legal troubles, and the difference I felt was awful. I felt claustrophobic and frustrated. I wasn't necessarily worried about the weight gain from lack of exercise, but more about my behaviours.

I felt more like the old me. I was more sedentary, I was hanging around the fridge and I was aware that I was trying to fix how I was feeling by shopping or eating more. It's scary how quickly you can fall back into those past patterns.

I knew I had to pull things back, so I made myself go to Barry's Bootcamp and do a class that I knew would push me. To begin with, I felt like I was back at beginner level and it was pretty depressing, but halfway through I felt the old spirit kick in and my energy came back. The change in my mood was genuinely shocking, and it reminded me just how important it is for me to keep my body moving and feeling strong.

The gym is so much about my mental health. I exercise because I like to feel fit and strong and I want good bone density and muscle mass. I exercise because I want to feel energetic and optimistic. I'm not there to try and get thin.

Be clear with yourself about your goals, so that you've got back-up at your fingertips when your motivation is low. It's so much easier to motivate yourself if you can say 'I exercise because I want more energy to run around with my kids' than to say 'I want to lose weight'. One is a motivation, the other is a downer!

Write your goals down now.

**I exercise because . . .**

## YOU CAN'T OUT-TRAIN A BAD DIET

Mental clarity is what keeps me on track with exercise, and I believe that comes from eating well. If I was trying to survive on two Twixes a day, or some god-awful processed-soup diet, I would soon falter because I wouldn't have the brain strength to keep me on track.

For me, feeling amazing means a combination of great food and consistent exercise. You will not get a body like an athlete if you're eating crap at the same time as working out, and you cannot outrun an inflammatory diet. In the old days, I went to the gym to give myself permission to eat cakes, but I know better now.

Also, you can't exercise like mad and still eat rubbish if you want to get lean. So many trainers have said to me over the years, 'Look, I know you're paying me to train you but losing weight is 90 per cent diet.'

Any personal trainer that takes fifty quid for an hour and doesn't also address your nutrition is stealing from you if you're trying to lose weight, because it is about diet too. Hopefully you will make better food decisions because you've balanced your hormones and you're in a good place anyway, but it's a two-way street.

## NOOTROPICS:
## WHEN YOU NEED AN ENERGY BOOST

If you're really struggling with motivation, and feel like you need more energy, I have had some great results with taking nootropics. Nootropics is one of those words that freaks people out a bit because it sounds really sciency, but they're basically supplements that give you more energy, better focus or even help you sleep (and yes, they are all legal!).

5-HTP and L-theanine are considered to be nootropics, along with the likes of ginseng and caffeine, so they're likely to be things you've already heard of. You can take them on their own or in formulas that blend several together, and I swear by them.

One of my favourite nootropic blends is a supplement that contains Alpha GPC, L-tyrosine, Acetyl-L-carnitine, Caffeine anhydrous, Lion's mane mushroom, Huperzine A, Rhodiola rosea, Ginkgo biloba and L-theanine (see page 243 for recommended suppliers).

If you're nervous about nootropics, try having a coffee before you train instead. Caffeine is one of the most-used nootropics and performance enhancers out there.

## WHY I TRAIN ON AN EMPTY STOMACH

For me, it's really important to work out on an empty stomach. You'll see in the two-week reset plan that I always recommend exercising first thing. It's going to be different for everyone, but I find it a lot easier to access energy if I exercise before I eat. I feel lighter and sharper. If I eat first, I don't feel like exercising because I can feel the food moving around inside me, and my body's moved into rest and digest mode.

I take my lead from hunter gatherers, who were able to switch on certain parts of their brains to make them more alert when they were in a fasted state. Also, if you train on an empty tummy your body will go into fat-burning mode quicker.

I like to exercise in the morning, but if I can't I'll extend my fast until I have got my workout in. Most people can run around 15k on residual energy before they need to refuel, so I don't bother with the pre-workout energy drinks. Like I said above, caffeine and other nootropics will give you a kick, but you really don't need to splash out on specialist drinks that cost a fortune.

At the end of the day, exercise starts in the brain, not a bottle. If you're not in the right frame of mind, whacking down an energy drink is not going to make you suddenly want to hit the gym.

It's worth saying that I feel really strongly about avoiding those sugary processed post-workout drinks, too.

When you're exercising, your muscles are working, and that means they start pumping out free radicals so that they can repair themselves. Your liver needs to process these free radicals after exercising. If you then have a packaged post-workout protein shake, on top of the free radicals, your liver has got to process the sweeteners and sugars from the shake, as well as the protein. So, your liver is actually doing ten times the amount of work it should be just to repair from the exercise. After exercising, I suggest you stick to the natural, healthy foods that your body can absorb easily.

Once I've worked out, I'll feel so much better and my entire day will take a different trajectory. Exercise can change my mood immediately. If I don't start the day well, I can easily go off track and start eating rubbish. But equally, I know that I can turn things around the following day. I know I can get control back easily because I've trained myself to, but I also want to be honest about the fact that I falter sometimes.

# EXERCISING FOR YOUR CYCLE

As any woman knows, there are times of the month where we have great energy, and times when we want to build a camp out of duvets in the cupboard under the stairs and stay there for several days.

Our hormones are a constantly evolving beast, especially if we're in perimenopause or menopause, so you need to work out the best ways to work out and eat according to your cycle. That's why period-tracker apps are so important.

If you check your app and you know you should be fine to exercise but you're too busy watching Phil and Holly, you should give yourself a gentle kick up the bum. But if you look and it clicks why you're feeling terrible and unmotivated, scale things back and go for a walk instead of a run, or do a bit of light exercise. Or if you feel really shit, do nothing on that day. You are allowed!

Over the years, I've learned to read my cycle and how it affects my energy levels really well, and here's what I recommend when it comes to exercising *with* your cycle, rather than against it.

## Menstruation: Days 1–5/6/7 (depending on your cycle)

Day one is the first day you bleed, and it's when your hormone levels are at their lowest, making you feel more tired. Yoga is a good option on these days, but as I'm not a fan I'll usually do some light weight sessions just to keep moving in a low-impact way. I avoid cardio at this time, and I won't exercise for more than forty minutes each day.

I ease up on the intermittent fasting during these days if I feel like I need to. Sometimes a drop in iron levels can affect your energy, and you may get cravings for sweet things. I prepare an avocado chocolate mousse in advance, which is full of antioxidants, to stop myself reaching for the Dairy Milk. Clams or a grass-fed rib-eye steak are also great to eat around this time due to their high iron levels.

## The follicular phase: Days 1–14

I tend to have a really brutal time on days three and four of my cycle. As a result, I will quite happily give myself a break and put my feet up. There is no point in me pushing myself and risking inflaming my already suffering body. But learn when you feel good and to work with your cycle. Hormone tracking apps can be a brilliant source of information on this.

If I'm feeling negative, a Wim Hof breathwork session can snap me out of it. The great thing is it requires zero physical effort. You can literally lie on your bed and breathe. You can find some of his exercises online, or on his app, and I give some instructions on page 186.

The good news is that during this follicular phase hormones start building again, so by day seven I'm back into running and plenty of leg exercises on a daily basis.

From day seven I'll go back to my usual intermittent fasting schedule.

## Ovulation: Day 14(ish)

Surging oestrogen can provide an increase in energy, giving you ovulation superpowers! This is a great time to challenge yourself by trying your first HIIT class, or trying to beat your 5K personal best.

Progesterone is low, meaning your pain tolerance is high, so you will recover more quickly from high-intensity exercise.

Again, I'll follow my usual intermittent-fasting schedule during these days.

## The luteal phase: Days 14–28

I still have a good amount of energy during this phase, so I continue to train. However, as I move beyond day 20 I go on longer, slower runs and keep to a steady fat-burning pace. I get out into nature as much as possible and use the daylight to increase my energy, as opposed to relying on coffee.

I'll still be following my regular intermittent-fasting schedule, and I will also add plenty of fresh cruciferous vegetables to my meals to help keep my hormones as balanced as possible before the big drop! You might crave carbs more in this phase and they will burn better as fuel in this high hormone phase as well as supporting serotonin levels. Go for whole food sources like root vegetables and avoid fried carbs.

# YOU DON'T NEED FANCY EQUIPMENT

Going to the gym is often a hurdle that we find hard to overcome. But there are plenty of great ways to exercise at home. When gyms closed due to lockdown, my kitchen became one of my favourite places to work out. When our food delivery arrives, I'll use the heavier bags to do a quick bit of arm toning. I hold the bags and curl my arms up for ten reps to do a spot of toning. It only takes about a minute, but it's all the small things that make a difference.

Exercise doesn't have to be complicated or require equipment. I sometimes do three sessions of one-minute straight planks a day. They take five minutes, and that's with a rest in between. They're great for tummy toning, they improve balance, lift your bum and help with spine strength (because what's going on inside our bodies is just as important as what's going on outside).

Or do ten squats while you wait for the kettle to boil – if you're drinking a lot of tea, this can really add up every day.

If you want to invest in a cheap bit of kit for home, you can get a medium-strength resistance band for about £20. Do twenty side-step squats followed by twenty standard squats, concentrating on your bum (while watching *This Morning*, obviously).

Make the most of what you have, and get creative.

## Home workout

These simple exercises can be done anywhere, adapted to household objects if you don't have weights or equipment.

### RUSSIAN TWIST

For this one you will need a heavy weight, such as a kettlebell or a melon (go for a watermelon if you can, they're huge!).

- Sit on the floor with your knees bent and your feet firmly on the floor.
- Lean back slightly, keeping your back straight, holding the weight out in front of you.
- Breathe out as you twist the weight to the left and hold for a few seconds.
- Breathe in as you come back to centre and hold for a few seconds.
- Breathe out as you twist the weight to the right and hold for a few seconds.

You get the gist! Rather than counting reps, I do this while playing a song – I'll do twists during the verses, and then rest during the chorus.

## SIT-UPS WITH WEIGHTS

---

- Holding the weight (or watermelon) in front of you, do as many sit-ups as you can manage.

If I've used a watermelon, I'll then blend it into a juice, because the magnesium it contains helps with both sleep and DOMS (Delayed Onset Muscle Soreness: basically, that horrible 'burn' you can feel the day after intense exercise).

---

# Work your butt!

Your bum has got loads of big muscles, which means that exercises that use your glutes help you to burn more fat. If you want to lose weight overall, even on your arms, working your glutes is going to help. Whenever I do a workout, I do extra bum reps (does that sound weird?) to increase fat burning. These are a couple of my favourites.

## SQUATS

---

- Stand with feet wider than hip-distance apart, lower your bum as low as you can, until you really feel your thighs engage. Then rise back up.

Repeat as many times as you can. When you feel that burn, say to yourself: 'Just five more!' That's how you get stronger.

---

**WALKING LUNGES**

- Stand up straight with your feet hip-width apart.

- Take a big step forward with your right leg, and lower your body as far as you can go. Keep your abdominal muscles tight (as if holding in a wee!) as that will help your balance.

- Then step forward with your left leg, and walk your lunges for as long as you can. I can't do this without music as the burn is too much!

Lunges are a great fat burner and I even like the ache afterwards. It's a feeling that gives me a boost of self-esteem.

# Weight training

Don't be afraid of weightlifting. A lot of women are fearful of weights, but I promise you, you are not going to end up looking like The Rock. Our bones get weaker when we lose oestrogen during the perimenopause, but if your body thinks your bones are under stress it will produce more bone cells, thus making you stronger. So lifting weights makes your body stressed enough that it actually builds more bone. Weak bone can lead to life-changing injuries, and frankly I want to be lifting weights whilst dancing to happy house well into my eighties.

Give kettlebells a go. They are amazing for toning and getting a full body workout. I use an 8kg bell these days, but as always, start light and build yourself up. There are some great tutorials on YouTube, and I recommend you start there as you need to be able to see the correct form and posture on an instructor. It's not something you should learn from a book.

## Join a team

Teamwork makes the dream work. Back in September 2018 I joined a netball team that some of my mates played for and I ended up having such a laugh. It was the first time I'd been on a court for about thirty years, and I didn't realise how strong my competitive streak was. As soon as we started playing, the competitive red mist descended and my psycho behaviour kicked in. But we had such a laugh it didn't even feel like exercise. There's also something lovely about being part of a team where you're all working together. I can't recommend it enough.

## Set a goal

Running the London Marathon was honestly a dream, even if it did give me massive blisters. One of the highlights was passing someone who was dressed up as a bottle of beer. I probably would have wrestled him to the ground and tried to drink him fifteen years ago.

I could never have imagined I would be able to do something that big, and when I think about the sense of achievement I felt when I crossed the finishing line and how proud Matthew and the boys were of me, it still makes me well up a bit.

I'm not suggesting for a minute that you sign up to run 26.2 bleedin' miles, but one of the great things about the lockdowns (and let's face it, there weren't many) was how many people did Couch to 5k. Even if you do kitchen to 2k when you haven't run for years, you'll feel so proud of yourself.

Find a goal that feels like it's a stretch, and make a plan for how you'll achieve it. You'll be amazed at what you can achieve and the self-confidence it will bring you.

## Rest

············

It's so important to allow your body to rest in between workouts – in the next section of the book I'm going to give you plenty of pointers about how best to do this.

Your body will not thank you for pushing it to its limits. You are not Mo Farah, there are no medals to win here! If I've had a big kettlebell session, I know I then need to get some oxygen to my poor muscles to help them recover. For me, the best way to do that is to have a cold bath or shower because as my body warms up afterwards, it gets flooded with oxygenated blood, thus speeding up recovery.

And please don't force yourself to exercise if you're feeling shit. A lot of women feel rubbish doing exercise while they're pre-menstrual, so don't drag yourself to the gym if you just want to go and cry in the corner.

If I have one of those days I'll sit in the sauna, or I'll hang off a pull-up bar and stretch my back out. Just something restorative and gentle. What I don't do is lie on the floor pretending I was going to do some sit-ups while eating jelly babies.

Slower exercises can be good for you. I always thought it was all or nothing with working out, but when I tried Pilates to help with pain in my right hip, I discovered just how dynamic and powerful slow movement can be. For years I thought of my body as a series of separate parts, but Pilates helped me to see my body as a whole. Every bit of your body talks to the other parts, so if something is out of kilter, it's going to have a knock-on effect on the rest of you. I still don't think yoga and I are ever going to see eye-to-eye, but I'm getting more open to the idea.

If you need any more incentive to exercise, just listen to what Dr Tam has to say about it:

'If you're exercising enough to raise your heart rate, you're going to be producing adrenaline and noradrenaline and endorphins, which are the body's natural painkillers. You're going to be activating your natural amino acids, which stimulate your brain. There are so many studies done that show exercise has a positive impact on your brain for different reasons. There's something called BDNF, which stands for brain derived neurotrophic factor. Cold exposure and saunas also really increase the expression of BDNF, which has an impact on your brain health. The healthier your brain is, the less prone you are to neurodegenerative disorders like Parkinson's, dementia, depression and addictive disorders. The younger you start looking after your brain, the better, and that can be done via diet, exercise and targeted supplementation.'

As if you need any more motivation. Get out there!

---

### DAVINIA'S FIVE MOVEMENT TAKEAWAYS

- Understand that exercise is a mood-boosting treat, not a punishment
- Get kitted out so you begin to think of yourself as an exerciser
- Make a commitment to walk every day for at least twenty minutes
- Work out your fat-burning zone – you should be able to talk at this pace
- Exercise your biggest muscles (your bum and thighs!) for maximum fat burning.

# REST

I honestly haven't seen enough information about the importance of rest when you are trying to live a healthy lifestyle. Like I said, everyone wants to know what I eat, or what my exercise regime looks like, but I never get asked about how much rest I take. And yet I have learned that this is one of the most important parts of living well. I get that many of you will be tempted to skip ahead to the two-week reset programme at this point – thinking *Rest?! Yeah, right, when will I have time for that?* But I promise you that rest is the missing piece of the puzzle for so many of us who want to look and feel better.

As much as we all want to live a calm, balanced life with plenty of time for relaxation, it doesn't always happen that way. We know we need good sleep and rest to truly feel well and happy, but when you've got kids, pets, other halves, jobs (the list goes on) it can be easy to find your wellbeing slipping to the bottom of your priority list. But I still factor in rest time, as what use am I going to be to anyone else if I'm burned out?

Resting doesn't need to look like going to a spa, or spending money on treatments or products. Of course if you want to treat yourself there are plenty of ways to splash out on ways to chill out but, to me, resting looks like deep breathing, going for a walk (on my own!) and listening to a podcast or audio book, or having a nap during the day if I need to.

I was going through a bit of a crazy time while I was writing this book. I was relocating, I was having to stay in London during the week (due to a complicated court case), and I was missing my family and the dogs so badly. I was also under huge financial pressure and, not surprisingly, my body, mind and sleep all suffered.

My physical and emotional energy were being drained on a daily basis, and because I was so stressed, the 'tryptophan steal' was rudely nicking all my serotonin.

Tryptophan is an amino acid that is converted to 5-HTP, and then eventually serotonin, but inflammation and stress cause tryptophan to be directed down an altered pathway, meaning there's less serotonin available to make us feel happy. When you find yourself really low from stress, this is worth knowing.

I also felt bloody miserable some days. I knew that if I didn't take good care of myself and allow myself to rest, I was going to end up very unwell. Eating well and exercising were not enough on their own. Actively making time to balance my nervous system by doing deep breathing and taking cold showers was every bit as important as what was on my plate, or how many miles I ran.

As soon as I made time to incorporate the things I'm going to talk about in this chapter, I remembered just how much of a difference they make to my everyday life.

## PLEASE BE KIND TO YOURSELF, YOU BLOODY DESERVE IT

Looking after myself has changed everything. It's made me more assertive and less vulnerable. I'm less likely to people-please and more likely to put my family and myself first. I have an inner confidence and self-esteem, which I didn't have before.

Taking care of my wellbeing has given me a lovely feeling that I'm doing something positive and I'm trying to influence my children in the best ways possible. I'm also trying to help people around me live longer, better and healthier lives by spreading the knowledge I've gained.

Even feeling better in clothes and having shinier hair make me feel better! My hair grows super-fast these days, and I'm sure that's down to having better nutrition.

I can get dressed a lot quicker because I don't have to think about fitting into stuff or trying to disguise bulges or hide my upper arms, or a belly that's hanging over my jeans. I can take an interest in fashion, and second-hand clothes look great on me too, so I don't have to spend fortunes on new ones, or comfort-shop.

This feeling of wellbeing is something I am determined to protect at all costs. I remember how it felt to be unhappy, bloated and miserable. So I understand that when I don't rest and restore myself, I am making it harder to feel my best, and that helps me make it a priority.

One of the first ways to rest is to give yourself a break from the constant barrage of stimulation from phones and computers. Stepping away from your phone for half an hour every now and again is essential, even for an Instagram addict like me. It's not easy, and I definitely don't do it every day, but I do notice a difference in my stress levels if I have some time out from social media.

When I was younger, I had terrible comparison-itis, and I admit I still often do it now. I call it 'compare and despair'. To keep my head straight, I won't buy certain magazines that I know have been airbrushed, and I won't follow certain accounts on Instagram that I know will make me feel insecure. You don't become your best self by following the accounts of people you think you're inferior to.

One of the best things I've done for my mental health was a social-media detox.

I edit the people I follow once a month, and the rule is that if they make me tut, they're culled. I know that sounds harsh, but I don't want to look at over-edited or over-filtered accounts filled with smugness. It's the reason I'm so honest in my posts. If I'm feeling crap, you're going to know about it. I want to stay real and happy. The more real and honest I am with myself and others, the stronger I feel.

I'm not claiming to be an expert in every area of health, but I've gone down some strange roads in my time and I've had to pull myself back from the brink. And I cannot tell you how much my life has turned around since I've finally found ways to keep my mind and body stable.

Taking steps towards managing stress, and finding ways to relax and restore, means less anxiety, which means fewer cravings and a healthier mental state, which makes it easier to make good decisions for myself all round.

A lot of the things I'm talking about in this section are really accessible and, best of all, free. Breathing is free, cold water is free, earthing is free and meditation is free. You really have *no* excuse not to give some of them a go.

## COLD-WATER THERAPY

When I first read about the phenomenon of cold-water therapy, I was desperate to try it, but oh my God, I was terrified. *Terrified*!

The theory behind cold-water therapy is that when you immerse yourself in cold water you trigger something called the 'mammalian diving reflex', which makes you breathe in really sharply. That kicks off the body's fight-or-flight response, so your adrenaline and cortisol kick in and make you feel really alert.

People take ice baths to kickstart this feeling, or they swim outside in all weathers, or they take cold showers. Does the idea of this freak you out? It did me!

Every reflex in my body wants to stay cosy and warm. Of course it does! I think there's an innate primal fear of the cold because it hurts and it's not nice. Even now that I've been using cold-water therapy for ages, I'm not going to lie, I don't love the feeling of it. I do it so I don't have to take anti-depressants, and I never quite believe people who say they love how it feels. It's *always* a shock to my system. I guess that's why it works!

So I fully resisted trying cold-water therapy, until I read that it could stimulate the vagus nerve and help regulate mood. I was still pretty unwilling to be uncomfortable, but that alone convinced me it would be worth trying.

After I came off the anti-depressants and decided it was time to properly look after myself, everything began with cold showers. I was still suffering with post-natal depression after having my fourth son, Jude, and I'd read about the mental-health benefits of a daily cold shower. I thought: *I want some of that. I don't want to feel low and unmotivated any more.*

Reading about cold-water exposure led me to the Dutch cold-water and breathwork genius, Wim Hof. His back story and work fascinated me. His wife tragically committed suicide due to depression in 1995, and he was left to bring up four kids alone. With his own mental health suffering, he started looking into the mechanics of cold exposure, and how as a race we've always been exposed to the cold, but nowadays we shy away from it.

Wim Hof started with yoga and cold-water therapy, and developed breathwork exercises which he believes helped him to build mental and physical resilience. Wim (I like to think we're on first-name terms!) developed and scientifically proved how his breathing technique and cold-water therapy helped rid him of disease and viruses, as well as depression. He was injected with *E. coli* endotoxin during one experiment and, without any medical intervention, he managed to activate his immune system to kill the virus. He, and his work, are mind-blowing and I massively recommend you seek him out if you're interested.

The final trigger for me to try cold-water therapy was when I learned that it can balance your hormones (for free!). I had nothing to lose, and better hormones and mental clarity to gain.

It is pretty hardcore to actually immerse yourself fully in cold water – either by wild swimming outdoors or by sitting in an ice bath. My advice is to start with a much more manageable technique of just turning your shower onto cold for a few seconds. You can then build this up to thirty seconds or a minute. I can't say I ever exactly look forward to it, but it is incredibly invigorating, and I really notice the difference if I skip it.

To maximise the effect of a cold-water shower, you can add a breathing technique. The ideal method is to breathe in for two to four seconds, and then out for five to eight seconds. That makes it more bearable. If you hum on the out breath, that's when you'll also activate the vagus nerve. Basically, once your body realises you're not actually dying, the parasympathetic system takes over to calm the situation and you get into a state of balance and optimisation (homeostasis), which creates a calming, cosy feeling thanks to your hormones, without tablets or alcohol. Winner.

I do get that it feels awful until you're used to it. I'm not saying for a minute that I loved it from day one. You're in there underneath the freezing water and it's horrible, horrible, horrible. Then all of a sudden, your body starts adapting and it's not so bad.

Try it for a few seconds to start with and build up from there. It's not a competition and you will know when you've had enough.

If your experience is anything like mine, one day you'll suddenly realise that you don't hate it as much as you did, and you can stay in the shower for longer and longer without having to force yourself. You might even (*whispers*) *enjoy* it.

It takes a lot of getting used to and you might have to get yourself psyched up. If you really can't face a cold shower at all, you could begin by submerging your face into a sink full of iced water to get yourself used to the feeling of the cold. Try that for a few mornings. Or if you sit in a really hot bath for twenty minutes first, you'll appreciate a cold shower much more.

Cold showers are an adaptogen, meaning they'll wake you in the morning and make you sleepy at night as your body regulates its temperature. If you need a cold shower to wake you up, it will do, but if your body knows it's night-time and it's time to wind down, your hormones will adjust accordingly.

Nature is so much cleverer than us. Cold-water therapy is so cheap and easy, it almost seems *too* simple.

Try having a cold shower at night and then get into a nice warm bed. There's nothing else like it.

Cold showers may be tough, but it's far worse having a hormonal imbalance and being pissed off. You don't even need to do it every day. Three times a week would produce huge benefits.

I've known people who have cried when they've first had cold showers, and I'm sure that's a release of hormones too. Personally, I felt better within a week of trying it.

If you need some more encouragement, here it is: having an ice-cold shower for ninety seconds = endorphins, better circulation, weight loss, stress relief, pain relief, muscle healing, increased alertness, anti-depressant qualities and an immunity boost. It also trains your brain and body to deal with stress better.

When I was still living in London, I'd sometimes pop along to a cryogenic chamber, which is an enclosed chamber that surrounds your body and immerses you in bitingly cold air for several minutes. Cryogenic chambers are super-convenient because you don't get wet, but there aren't any around where I live now, so I've gone totally down the DIY route.

I've been wild swimming (which is very on-trend right now – it basically means leaping into a lake) in the Serpentine in London, as well as in some lakes and rivers up north. It's tricky to take that first step, but once you do, you won't look back. I'm also a huge fan of swimming in the sea, which is obviously a lot nicer if you're in a hot country. I find sea swimming really grounding, and if I feel myself drifting off into the future and worrying about what's to come, something about wild swimming helps to bring me back to the now and 'keep it in the day', as they say in AA.

## BREATHWORK

It's easy to find our emotions overwhelming, and when mine started coming back after I stopped taking anti-depressants, I began to really *feel* everything again, which made me nervous at times. I wanted to find a way to calm myself down that didn't send me back into my old addictive patterns. And that's where Wim Hof's breathwork came in.

Wim's experience has been backed up by scientific evidence that demonstrates how breathwork can alter the body's chemical imbalances using oxygen and $CO_2$, and thus heal, reduce inflammation at a cellular level and calm the mind.

Even though as we know I'm not into woo-woo, I love how Wim mixes science with spirituality and makes it so accessible. I have trouble accepting anything airy-fairy, and therefore find it hard to commit to anything that's too out-there. But what he does makes sense to me, and it did even in the beginning, before I delved deep into the biohacking world.

You can download his app for free and give it a go, and I would highly recommend it if you fancy getting high off your own supply. Or I've given a simplified version below if you want to try that first.

The first time I tried his breathing exercises, I did three rounds of breathing in for longer than I breathed out, and after two rounds I got this weird tingly feeling and I lost my sense of time and space. I'm not kidding! It was totally trippy.

## BREATHWORK EXERCISE

As mentioned above, breathwork can make you feel quite trippy, so please do not attempt any kind of breathwork while driving or in any other situation where you need to concentrate. I recommend you do this exercise sitting down.

- Take thirty deep breaths in through the mouth to a count of two, and out for the count of one. You're trying to get as much oxygen into your bloodstream as possible, and this is the bit where you may feel a bit lightheaded.

- Once your blood is oxygenated, take a breath and hold it for as long as you can. When you can't hold it for any longer, breathe out, and then pause, with all the air out of your lungs, for ten seconds.

You build up the length of time you can hold your breath each time, and eventually you'll be able to hold a single breath for two or three minutes – or maybe even longer – with no effort. Each time you practise, you're lowering your $CO_2$ level right down, which enables you to hold the breath for longer.

---

I went to a talk with Wim at the Round House in Camden, and the irony of me deep-breathing in a place where I used to party like a lunatic was not lost on me. The science behind what Wim does is fascinating, however.

It's about time his method went super-mainstream. The benefits to your body and mind are far beyond anything I've encountered. It's helped me to engage in a chilled-out activity which still gives a deep cardio workout (yep, it also does that for you) and expands the mind, resulting in clearer thinking and focus.

I'm not someone who loves meditation – I have tried it and feel like I should take it up again, but (much like yoga) it just doesn't rock my world. Yet sitting still and focusing on this breathwork exercise acts a bit like meditation for me.

I feel a chemical shift in my head and I get lights in my eyes and it really is quite trippy. I like to see real results fast and this only takes five minutes. With transcendental meditation you need to do twenty minutes in the morning and evening, and that just never feels achievable for me, to be honest.

I feel like I'm the only woman on the planet who doesn't love yoga and meditation and I hate missing out. Maybe I'm missing the yoga and meditation gene?

## HOT STUFF

It's not just cold therapy that's good for you. Heat is also an amazing way to restore the body to its optimum. You can just take a nice hot bath, perhaps with a blast of cold shower afterwards. But I am a big fan of taking heat therapy up a notch by using infra-red saunas.

The human race has sweated for ever, and it's so good for you. In my opinion, we don't sweat enough these days. Any kind of sauna is good for you, but I prefer infra-red over the more traditional steam saunas.

The main difference between the two is that infra-red uses light to heat the body from within, whereas traditional saunas use air to heat the body from the outside.

It's claimed that the heat from infra-red saunas penetrates the skin more deeply, leading to a larger elimination of toxins. As soon as I heard that, I was sold.

I bought my own infra-red sauna for £140 on Amazon and I swear, it's one of the best investments I've ever made.

Saunas really help me with cravings, so I like to have them very regularly. Which is why, if you look at some of my Instagram videos, you'll see me looking like a floating head wearing a massive silver puffa jacket while I'm enjoying my home sauna.

Studies suggest that infra-red saunas:

- Improve your mood and have an anti-depressant effect

- Stimulate lymph flow via sweat (our all-important lymphatic system helps to remove waste and toxins from our bodily tissues)

- Get your bowels moving as the muscles in your abdomen relax

- Help with weight loss

- Lessen fatigue

- Increase relaxation

- Reduce feelings of frustration and anxiety

- Stimulate your mitochondria, so you produce more energy.

The way they help with weight loss is that, as fats break down, the toxins stored inside the fat cells are released into your bloodstream. You can remove them by sweating them out in a sauna. If you don't remove the toxins, they will be reabsorbed into your body. And no one wants that.

When you're in any sauna, infra-red or not, your heart rate increases, your blood vessels dilate and you begin to sweat more, which in turn causes an increase in blood circulation. I recorded my heartbeat during one of my very early sessions, and it went up to 130BPM, which is equivalent to a 5k jog. I felt so smug.

I look utterly ridiculous in my mini sauna and Matthew and the kids find it hilarious, but it's worth the mickey-taking because I feel so good afterwards. If I sit in it for forty minutes watching TV, it lifts my mood and helps with water retention.

The reason saunas help with mental health (and why I sleep so well afterwards) is because having regular saunas lowers cortisol levels. If your cortisol levels are too high, you don't produce enough serotonin (which we all know by now is the happy hormone) because the thieving cortisol does a runner with it. When your cortisol lowers, your serotonin levels go up and that helps you feel more relaxed. It's even said to be able to induce a state of meditation, but I am yet to experience that in my sauna. Maybe because half the time when I'm zipped up and sweating the kids are shouting to ask what time dinner is.

I don't know if it's a detox thing and it helps my liver, which then helps my gut, which in turn helps my brain because they're so closely connected. But that's my hypothesis, anyway.

Every now and again I take a high dose of niacin (also known as vitamin B3) before I have a sauna, which is said to be a brilliant way to get rid of cravings that are caused by low mood and depression. Make sure you buy the flush version, as opposed to the non-flush, because there is evidence that the non-flush version doesn't actually provide the body with much niacin, making it pretty ineffective. Bill W., who is one of the founders of AA, was known to use niacin to help with alcohol cravings, and I think it's fair to say he knew his stuff.

But please tread carefully and don't go hell for leather. I know someone who bought her dad the same sauna as I've got. She also bought him some niacin but gave him strict instructions not to use it straight away, so he could give his body time to get used to the effects of the sauna first. She also told him not to take the niacin the day after he'd been drinking. Believe me, you do not want to take niacin with a hangover. You'll feel like you're about to pass out, because the effects will be amplified due to the increased amount of toxins in your body.

Now, her dad isn't one of those people who listens to instructions very carefully, and even if he does, he'll do what he wants anyway.

He got his sauna all set up, whacked it up to 90 degrees (bearing in mind he hadn't been in a sauna for years) and, just to top things off, he took some niacin for the first time ever. You know, just to *really* go for it. Did I mention he'd also been drinking the night before?

He was in the sauna for two minutes before he came stumbling downstairs in his dressing gown, bright red in the face, saying he 'felt a bit funny, like he might pass out'. I don't know if any of you tried poppers in your youth (and if you haven't, really, really don't), but if you're not used to niacin, or you're taking it after drinking alcohol, it produces a similar feeling. You basically go bright red and feel like your head might explode.

Thankfully the dodgy feeling (and his bright red face) calmed down within a few minutes, but there's a good lesson in there. Yes, saunas are great for detoxing, weight loss and mental health, but take things slowly to begin with. It's not a 'who can get the hottest' competition. Give your body a chance to understand what's going on.

Quite often, I'll go straight from the sauna into a really cold bath, and I'm basically doing my own at-home cryo protocol. The alternation in hot and cold is great for your hormones.

You can do the same thing with a hot and cold shower, so I'm not suggesting that everyone pops out and buys themselves a sauna, but if you really want one, why not ask people to contribute for your next birthday or Christmas? I swear, you'll never regret it.

## SPIKE MAT

My spike mat (aka an acupressure mat) is also one of the best things I've ever bought. These are foam mats with little spikes all over them – almost like a bed of nails – which you lie on. And they work on the same acupressure principles, by stimulating blood flow and helping you to enter a deep state of relaxation. If you're feeling sceptical, I don't blame you. It seemed a bit nuts to me at first, but enough people had recommended it that I thought it was worth the twenty-quid investment. (You can buy more expensive ones, but the basic principle is the same, so I don't see the point.)

I cannot recommend it enough. Supposedly a spike mat can help reduce stress, eliminate headaches, increase blood flow and circulation, positively affect the nervous and immune systems, help muscles recover faster after exercise, and increase energy levels. For twenty bloody quid!

You lie on the mat either with bare skin or with a light T-shirt on – it depends how sensitive your skin is. At first it can feel pretty weird, and a little uncomfortable, but go with it and you'll find that your body relaxes into the sensation. In fact, it feels really good, sort of like scratching an itch! When you get up from the mat, you can almost feel the blood flowing more energetically around the body.

As I've said, I'm not someone who's great at meditation or just sitting completely still, so it's not like I lie on this mat in a state of perfect Zen silence. To be honest, I'm usually watching Netflix or doing stuff on my phone at the same time. But I still feel the benefits afterwards, and I really notice how much it helps with my sleep, too.

## GET GROUNDED

Earthing, also known as grounding, consists of really simple techniques that electronically reconnect you to the earth's electrons (bear with me). I realise that, considering I shun woo-woo, earthing sounds a bit out-there for me. But it's actually very science-based, and it really works. Because at the end of the day, our bodies are electric. Think about when someone's heart stops and they pump them with electricity to try to get it going again.

Our cells conduct electrical currents, and electricity enables the nervous system to send signals throughout the body and to the brain, which makes it possible for us to move, think and feel.

The earth is a powerful source of electricity, which can be accessed via barefoot exposure, even on concrete. If you stand outside on the earth, the theory goes, because it's a magnetic field it grounds you and fills you with energy.

It costs nothing to take your shoes and socks off and walk around on the grass for half an hour, and you'll be doing your body and mind a lot of good. It conducts a current that can balance your hormones and bring inflammation right down for absolutely no cost at all. And you don't have to be on a beach in Barbados: you can literally do it anywhere.

Go barefoot whenever possible. Wherever you are in the

world, the earth emits a 7.38-hertz frequency, and the natural magnetic frequency assists with our circadian rhythm (our natural sleep cycle) and the absorption of negativity-charged free electrons, which can mitigate stress.

Earthing also lifts your mood and aids recovery after exercise. The Tour de France teams use earthing mats in bed to recover faster for the next day of gruelling cycling, so if you don't fancy walking around in the cold, you can get your own for around forty quid.

I know all this might sound a bit mad, but it's free and you can do it right now, so I reckon it's worth a try. And I have noticed a real difference when I make an effort to ground regularly.

## BEAUTY HACKS

I am not much of a one for facials or other treatments that are going to take up loads of my time, but I really notice that I feel uplifted mood-wise when I feel good about how I look. And when I feel good about myself, I'm less inclined to give in to cravings or any other destructive behaviours. So I'm all about the little hacks that make me feel my best, without having to book an appointment or travel to a clinic. I think we all know that the best beauty tip is to feel good about yourself. But a few beauty tricks can really help you out, and these are some of my favourites – do check with a dermatologist first though. Engaging in a bit of self-care is a great way to unwind, too.

# Natural skincare

I have definitely noticed a difference in my skin since I started exercising and eating more healthily. I don't get as many breakouts, and even though I'm getting older I'm doing all right for lines and wrinkles. I would put that down to plenty of vitamin C drops and pasture-raised collagen supplements on top of a good diet.

Collagen is incredible for your skin. I take it as a pure powder (never pre-mixed), a teaspoon dissolved in water or a hot drink – I aim for about six grams a day, so that's about three teaspoons overall. Always go for the most natural supplements or powder you can find, and make sure powders are unsweetened (sugar finds its way into *everything*). My preferred brands are at the back of the book.

I also take astaxanthin supplements, which are amazing for your skin. This a reddish dye (a keto-carotinoid, if you want to get scientific about it) produced by green algae. It's the same stuff that makes lobsters red and flamingos pink! It helps improve blood pressure, cholesterol, etc., and it's great for the skin. I've been told that it prevents wrinkles and sun damage, and I really notice the difference when I take it. I always dose up before holidays, and in the summer when I'm going to be out in the sun.

I definitely look after my skin better than I did when I was in my twenties and thirties. I used to wear a lot more make-up back in the day, to hide my hangovers, and I'd often fall asleep without even bothering to wash my face.

Because I live a pretty healthy lifestyle these days, I sometimes take my good skin for granted. But I really saw the difference skincare can make when I was going through a very stressful time. I was involved in an emotionally draining court case and had also moved to Lancashire after several months in Spain. One of the boys was still at school in London, so I was constantly travelling between Lancashire and London and staying in a rented apartment in London, and everything got out of sync. That was the first time I realised just how essential taking care of your skin is.

I was rushing around so much, my skincare routine fell by the wayside and I was washing my face with shampoo while I was in the shower (I know!). I wasn't cleansing properly or using any of my usual oils or creams, and my skin felt and looked awful. I definitely learned my lesson.

If I have any breakouts, I will dry out my skin with some cheap and very basic baking soda, which I mix with water and rub over my face. I'll then add a spritz of hydrogen peroxide 3–6 per cent (this is just oxygenated water, it's not bleach!) that I've decanted into a water spray. I spritz that onto my face until the baking soda fizzes a little bit. If you have sensitive skin, this might be a bit much, so do a small patch test first.

After the treatment, I'll wash my face thoroughly with a gentle face wash, before I add a face oil (see the shopping list at the back of the book for my favourite brands).

I try to go as natural as possible with skincare and cosmetics, because anything you put on your face and body is going to have to be processed through your liver. I have learned that upping the toxic load on my liver will steal energy from me, and I want as much energy as I can possibly get, for my muscles and my brain.

I use organic shampoo and conditioner, and I spray perfume on my hair instead of my skin, where it won't be absorbed into the body. Our skin is our biggest organ, so we need to treat it kindly and not overload it with highly perfumed, toxic creams.

## Get rid of your scented candles!

Speaking of scent, this isn't strictly a beauty tip, but I think it fits here because so often when we think of self-care and beauty we think: *ooh, run a bath, light a lovely candle and relax.* But it's important to understand that many artificially perfumed candles are full of toxins that the body can absorb.

In addition, perfumes (even some natural ones like lavender) can act as endocrine disruptors, which means they interfere with the body's hormonal systems. Animal studies have linked endocrine disruptors to adverse effects, including imbalance of homeostasis, i.e. the normal functioning of our bodies. I don't want to mess up my hormones. I've got enough going on.

So that's the reason I don't use candles, unless I know they're completely natural and made from pure beeswax. There's one particular, very trendy brand that charges nearly fifty pounds for a small candle that contains petroleum. When you burn these candles, you're literally burning petroleum in your home, and I'm not spending a fortune to inhale more toxins.

There's a brilliant documentary on Netflix called *Scent* that I would really recommend you watch. It's all about the toxic additives in everything from kids' clothes to cosmetics.

As we age, it's harder for our bodies to detox, and I want to give myself the best chance I can of living to a ripe old age. Our liver has to detoxify the toxins from these candles and cleaning products when it really should be busy processing everyday toxins we can't avoid. Your body has to detox toxins as a priority because they're the most immediate threat, and only then can it start getting rid of fat. I believe if your body contains too many toxins you're bound to put on weight, and I am not getting fat for the sake of a fancy-smelling candle.

# White teeth hack

I usually use a plain organic toothpaste, but sometimes the glamour puss in me wants to feel more fabulous and have a sparkling white smile.

I had my teeth professionally whitened about twenty years ago and it was bloody agony afterwards, and I never want to go through that again, so I've come up with my own DIY whitening regime. Do check with your dentist before taking these steps, but I have been doing this for decades without any problems.

This treatment is for your teeth, not your gums. So avoid putting it on your gums, and avoid scrubbing the treatment, just leave it on the teeth without brushing.

If you're still worried this sounds too harsh, a gentler alternative is to mix together a tablespoon of coconut oil with a quarter teaspoon of activated charcoal powder. Apply to the teeth, leave for five minutes, rinse out and brush as normal.

**Step 1** Once a month, I dip my toothbrush in some hydrogen peroxide 6% 20 vols, which sounds scary but is just oxygenated water. I then add baking soda to my toothbrush to form a paste. I coat my teeth and leave it to fizz for 30–40 seconds, and then spit it out.

**Step 2** I remember my hairdresser telling me about Pearl Drops pink toothpaste, which works on the same basis as a colour-adjust shampoo. If your hair is yellow and brassy, you put a purple or bright-pink shampoo on it, which tones the yellow down to a whiter-based cool blonde. This toothpaste does the same for yellow teeth and I love it when I've overdone the coffee drinking.

**Step 3** Follow the whole process up by brushing your teeth with Sensodyne toothpaste, which helps rebuild enamel.

You need to really look after your teeth and your mouth. The mouth is the beginning of the gut and contains tons of microbiomes. It's basically your first line of defence.

## Cellulite

I have got cellulite on my legs, and it's definitely genetic. My mum was tiny but she had it too, and so did my grandmother, who was always on a diet and battled with her weight. Cellulite is a connective-tissue issue, not a fat issue, so even really slim people get it.

No matter your size, it can be a constant 'companion', but it feels so unfair. I exercise like a beast and eat well, yet it's still there, waving at me as I stand in the shower. No matter how hard I train or how lean I get, I always seem to have that damn puckering on the back of my thighs.

I've tried lotions and potions, and while some may have helped a bit because of the amount of time you have to spend massaging them in, I realised that I would be better off using a bit of kit I already owned.

I was using my spike mat one day to soothe my stiff back and shoulders, when I realised that its main job was to increase blood flow and circulation. It was a lightbulb moment where I thought: *If I could do that in the areas where I have cellulite, maybe I could make the connective tissue healthier by increasing the amount of oxygen in that area?*

I lay on my spike mat for twenty minutes and popped the spike pillow under my bum and thigh area, and I repeated the process several times a week.

I am also taking DIM (Diindolylmethane, to give it its full name). It's a supplement which is made up of a chemical called indole-3-carbinol, which is formed in our bodies and also found in cruciferous vegetables, like cabbage and broccoli. It's said to break down excess recirculating oestrogen and help with PMT and menopause symptoms. Because it helps to balance hormones, it's thought to minimise the effects of excess oestrogen, one of which is cellulite.

I take it alongside a supplement called phosphatidylcholine, which is really good for the brain, liver, cell membrane support and (because it's a fat emulsifier) cellulite. It also supports collagen production. The weaker the collagen and connective tissues are, the looser the skin is, and therefore the more obvious cellulite becomes.

I'm attacking my cellulite from both the inside and now the outside, and while I'm not quite cellulite-free yet, it's definitely helping, and I can see the effects. It took about three weeks to see a difference, so be patient!

## BATHS (THE WARM KIND)

I love a relaxing hot bath, but in a bid to steer clear of toxins I go as natural as possible with what I put in it. With all of these baths I recommend you drink a large glass of water while you're in the bath – add a squeeze of lemon juice and a pinch of sea salt to replace the electrolytes.

**Epsom salt bath** Epsom salts are amazing because your body will absorb the natural magnesium, which we need for sleep and stress management, and make you feel more relaxed. I use loads (about two cupfuls) in the bath and then I'll sit in the bath for at least twenty-five minutes to get the full benefit.

**Detox bath**  Another great detox bath is where you add a cup of baking soda, a third of a cup of hydrogen peroxide and a cup of bentonite clay, which draws impurities out of your system. Sit in the bath for about twenty-five minutes to allow it all to work. Do check with a doctor before trying a detox bath.

**Apple cider vinegar bath**  And finally (bear with me on this one because I know it can smell a bit dodgy), apple cider vinegar is brilliant for detoxing and relaxing your joints. I know it's not exactly Chanel No. 5 bath oil, but it will probably do you a lot more good. You can always add some essential oils to mask the chip-shop smell!

## SLEEP

Years of drinking and hardcore medications had messed up my sleep patterns, and as I started to pay attention to my body I became very aware that when I was tired I comfort-ate much more. Your body's natural response to being tired is to crave high-fat, high-sugar, fast-energy snacks.

Studies have shown that a lack of sleep can affect hunger hormones, which increase your appetite and cortisol levels, and that impacts how you store weight.

I was in a vicious cycle of sleeping badly and then wanting to binge on sugar, and sleeping badly the next night as a result. And so it went on. I didn't want to be overweight and exhausted.

Unstable blood-glucose levels make it more difficult to fall asleep and stay asleep, and mine were all over the place. If you don't get enough sleep, your body can't regulate your blood glucose as well, so you end up with higher levels, hence you crave more.

I had to break the cycle, and as I was still reliant on food to make me feel 'good', I tackled my sleep first. I didn't know about the gut–brain relationship back then, and even though I could feel what I ate and its effects on me, I wasn't *quite* ready to cut out takeaways and chocolate.

Sleeping should be one of those things that's second nature, but life gets in the way. We go on holiday, we go through really stressful times, or from nowhere we start to suffer with anxiety. Don't give yourself a hard time about it and berate yourself for not sleeping properly, because you'll only make things worse. Getting good sleep is just another habit (check out the section on habits in the 'Mood' chapter for more info).

It's also paramount that you have a decent mattress. All the adverts are right: you really do spend a third of your life in bed, and I think the bigger the bed, the better. I can't handle having contact with another human while I'm trying to sleep.

I can't tell you how nice it is to be able to sleep without wine or tablets now. When I was drinking, I wasn't *really* sleeping, because alcohol affects the quality of your sleep. It's fake sleep because you usually just pass out. I'd always wake up feeling really sluggish because I was getting a bit of deep sleep but I was hardly getting any REM (Rapid Eye Movement) sleep, which is the restorative type our bodies need.

Healthy brains that don't have plentiful carb stores go into ketosis (fat-burning mode) in REM, and it's also when the brain repairs itself. When you're in REM you produce deuterium-depleted water, which is a massive antioxidant that clears our free radicals (unstable atoms that can harm cells). So, if you're falling asleep drunk, not only are you filling yourself up with toxins, you're also not then detoxing them (again, no drinking judgement here!).

I cannot stress enough that sleep is the most important biohack, and being able to quantify and track it is paramount for your future health. I use an Oura ring these days and I love to see how the protocols I use increase my REM sleep and help me feel better in every way.

It took me a little bit of time to work out what suited me sleep wise, and you may have to do the same, but the pay-off is so worth it. I still have the odd bad night, like everyone else, but if I wake up at 3 a.m. or 4 a.m. I feel calmer just knowing that I have resources to help me get back to sleep faster.

I'm definitely less of a nightmare on the school run now I sleep better. Well, sometimes.

One of the first things I did to try and improve my sleep was to learn the basics of 'sleep hygiene', and my top tips are:

- Don't eat late because digestion can interfere with sleep
- Don't do high-intensity exercise later in the evening, as it can be too stimulating
- Allow yourself thirty minutes (device-free!) wind-down time before bed
- Have a set pre-bedtime routine, whether that's meditating, stretching or reading
- Dim your lights before bed and avoid bright overhead lights
- Go to bed and wake up at the same time each day. Yes, even at weekends. No lie-ins allowed! A fluctuating schedule plays havoc with your sleep rhythm
- Make sure your bedroom isn't too warm. Our body

temperature naturally drops at night, to let us know it's time to rest. If you keep your bedroom cool, you're reinforcing that message to your body, so you should drop off more easily. Temperatures between 60 and 68 degrees Fahrenheit also increase production of our sleep hormone, melatonin, which is said to be anti-ageing!

- Ditch the illuminated alarm clock. The light will keep you awake, and tracking the hours you lie awake is going to make you more stressed and unable to sleep. Similarly, checking your phone in the middle of the night will wake you up completely. Keep a night light in the bathroom to avoid blue lights for middle-of-the-night trips.

You've got to have a good routine if possible. Having said that, I am human and I'm totally guilty of lying in bed scrolling through Instagram at stupid o'clock when I should be sleeping. I just try and keep it to the bare minimum.

## UNDERSTAND THE POWER OF LIGHT

One of the most important pieces of the puzzle when it came to improving my sleep was understanding the effect of light on our bodies. In the days before artificial lighting and alarm clocks, our ancestors went to sleep when it was dark and woke when it was light. We have evolved so that our skin absorbs light (particularly through our eyelids), and then sends signals to our brains to say that it must be time to get up. And when it's dark, the messages to the brain tell the body it's time to sleep.

This means if your room is too light and you've got a lot of bare skin on show, your body will send a message to the brain that it's time to get up, even if it's 5 a.m. You've probably noticed yourself that you naturally wake up earlier in the summer than in the winter: it's what we've evolved to do.

So one very simple and immediate hack for better sleep is to make your room as dark as possible. Blackout blinds are a must. I've just bought a few on Amazon and they were so cheap. If you can't have a blackout blind, you really need an eye mask, and to cover yourself up with light, loose clothing so that you're not exposing too much skin to the light.

Obviously, we should be lively during the day and want to sleep at night, but things like jetlag, partying, working irregular hours and artificial light can send it all haywire.

Tim Gray, aka @Timbiohacker, taught me a lot about sleep and has been an invaluable part of my wellness journey (even writing 'wellness journey' feels ridiculous). He's always on hand to answer questions or tell me about the latest amazing gadget. He's been in that world a lot longer than I have and I trust his impartial advice and infinite wisdom on all things biohacky. He comes up with some mad ideas sometimes, but I embrace them. He was the first to introduce me to the magical work of 'blue blocking glasses', which quickly changed my sleep patterns for the better.

The science behind these glasses is that blue light from phones, computers and televisions knackers your sleep by ruining melatonin production. Blue light tells your body it's time to get up, and of course that's an issue if it's night-time. An excess of blue light can have negative side effects such as migraines, headaches and anxiety. It also plays havoc with your hormones.

If you wear blue blocking glasses, they allow you to see screens without experiencing the effects of the damaging blue light. I find they are great if I'm stuck indoors with the lights on or staring at at a screen. I wear mine a lot, and I also make sure I get plenty of sunlight, which helps to regulate your circadian rhythm (more hormone balancing), which is your natural internal sleep/wake pattern. If you worry about not getting enough natural light during the day, I would recommend getting a SAD lamp to help keep your levels up.

If you really struggle with sleep, I suggest getting the blue blocking glasses with red or orange lenses, which mimic the end of daylight, and not watching TV before bed to give yourself the greatest chance of nodding off. I'm only able to watch TV before bed because I've trained myself to be able to relax when it's on, but obviously it can be very stimulating.

I generally put my glasses on as soon as it starts to get dark and the electric lights come on. I look like Deirdre Barlow in them, but you have to suffer for your health. I've got clear ones now, because the orange-tinted ones ruined Netflix for me a bit. They skew the colour and I like to be able to see what colour people's outfits and highlights are.

I like to have a certain amount of time to unwind with Matthew before bed, so I do my Zen time with him next to me, which usually involves me lying on a spike mat with my blue blocking glasses on, watching Netflix. Hot.

## SUPPLEMENTS FOR SLEEP

These days I very rarely have trouble sleeping as my body feels balanced, but everyone has times when it's harder to drift off than others.

I take things on a night-by-night basis depending on how I'm feeling. I think we all get a sense of whether or not we're going to sleep well as soon as our head hits the pillow. If I know I need to hack into my mood in order to be in a good place the next day, I'll add in 5-HTP.

Here are a few of the supplements that help me to fall asleep more easily. Try these out, but also be the expert on yourself and pay attention to how you feel after taking anything new. For example, I have heard so much about how great CBD oil is for sleep, but it's never done anything in particular for me. And I've also heard from some medical professionals that CBD isn't great for everyone – supposedly it is great if you're anxious, but not so good if you're depressed.

- **Magnesium** You can either take 300mg of magnesium glycinate before bed, or just use some Epsom salts in bath, and let the magnesium be absorbed through your skin – it's the biggest organ in your body after all.

- **Melatonin** This is only available on prescription in the UK. It's better than sleeping pills as it's a naturally occurring hormone in your body, so you don't get that groggy feeling afterwards. To trigger your own natural melatonin production, I recommend concentrated cherry juice or bananas.

- **GABA** As mentioned before, GABA is a naturally occurring amino acid that is made in the brain and can also be taken in supplement form. As well as improving mood and reducing anxiety, it can also help with sleep.

- **L-theanine** As explained earlier, this is an amino acid which you take in tablet form or as a powder. Because it lowers anxiety and chills you out, it can help with sleep, particularly if your mind is racing. The combinations with lemon balm work best.

- **Trytophan and 5-HTP** I find these really helpful as both of these ingredients produce melatonin in the body. The supplement I take also contains vitamin B6 and zinc, which converts them to serotonin. An all-round winner. However, you should not take these if you are on anti-depressant medications as it can cause serotonin syndrome.

---

### DAVINIA'S FIVE REST TAKEAWAYS

- Prioritise rest as an essential (not optional!) part of a healthy lifestyle
- Try cold showers to regulate hormones and boost mood
- Try using heat therapy, with baths or saunas
- Find natural beauty treatments, and avoid artificial fragrances
- Develop good sleep hygiene.

# TWO-WEEK RESET PROGRAMME

OK, now comes the fun bit – we're going to get cracking!

I've armed you with loads of information, and you can go back and reference all the information in this book at any time, so I don't want any excuses. Here's where we get to put everything into action.

Fast-forward and picture your happy, healthy, future self. Like what you see? Put in the work, and we can get you there. Remember to check with your doctor before embarking on radical changes to your fitness and diet regime.

The key things I've already taught you for these first two weeks are:

• How to read labels
• How to intermittent-fast safely

209

- How to find out what your trigger foods are
- How to make delicious fatty coffee
- How to use hot and cold therapy
- How to get back into exercise.

All of these things will be invaluable over the next couple of weeks.

## KEEP YOUR
## MOOD AND FOOD DIARY GOING

I cannot emphasise enough how important your mood and food diary is going to be to you. I still write one now if I know I'm feeling a bit off and I want to get to the bottom of what's going on. I also find it really cathartic to jot down how I'm feeling, rather than stewing and getting angry and resentful.

Hands up, I used to think journalling was bollocks, but you can't argue with something that works, can you? Buy yourself a notebook or diary and a pen you love – because stationery shopping is bloody brilliant – and get busy.

You need to write down everything you eat. Always remember that classic saying: if you bite it, write it.

## SOME IMPORTANT POINTS

First off, I just want to say that it took me a good three years of experimenting, tons of investigating and lots of trial and error before I found a plan that really worked for me, and this is how I get back on track. What took me years can take you two weeks.

This is the actual reset I do myself if I fall off the wagon, so I know it's doable and I know it works. I would never expect anyone to try something I hadn't done numerous times myself with fantastic, fast results. But I'm not going to lie, it's a little hardcore.

If it feels a bit too much to take on all at once, feel free take it as slowly as you want. But I have to say that the more of the suggested steps you do at once, the greater the benefit to you, and you will reset yourself quicker. Personally, I like short, sharp shocks and getting through the pain barrier as quickly as possible, but I appreciate that we're all different.

I am very aware that the plan may feel overwhelming when you first look at it, or you may have social commitments, so you may want to dip your toe in and cherry-pick *some* of the things on the plan before you embrace it as a whole. You may find you don't like the taste of celery juice, or kombucha isn't for you. Take what you want from it and leave the rest, and do it at your own pace. (*Whisper* No one is going to know apart from you.)

Over the years, I've become an expert when it comes to my body, and now it's time for you to become your own expert (of your body, not mine. That would be weird).

By following this plan and paying attention to how you feel, you will learn things like how your body responds to certain foods, and whether you adore breathwork for relaxation or prefer a long bath. Hopefully it's going to be one of the most exciting learning curves you've ever experienced.

You'll be surprised just how much you're going to achieve by doing this reset. You're going to be balancing your hormones with the hot and cold showers, you're going to be repopulating your gut with good bacteria thanks to the food you're eating, and you're giving your body a chance to have a bloody good rest and repair.

## Ditch the junk today

The number-one most important thing you have to do before you begin this plan is a kitchen detox. I know it will be hard, but please box up anything that contains refined sugars and inflammatory oils because they are no longer a part of your diet. They lower your mood and increase hunger, and we want to do the opposite.

You can always pass them on to friends or donate them to a food bank so they don't go to waste.

I promise you, getting rid of the inflammatory foods is the kindest thing you can do for yourself right now. You're stripping away temptation and from now on you only put things that make you feel good in your body (and yes, that does mean the odd glass of red wine or chocolate mousse).

Please don't panic and think you're not taking in enough nutrition during the day on this plan. We know I count chemicals and not calories, but just as an example, a fatty coffee with one tablespoon of MCT oil will provide you with 115 calories and 14g of fat, and I have two tablespoons so I'm having 230 calories per MCT coffee, Matcha tea or bone broth, plus I'm feeding my brain with great stuff at the same time. And you will be eating hearty, nutritionally dense, delicious meals every night, as well as snacks, so you will not be short of food.

If any of the daytime meals during the first week of the plan are tricky because you work in an office or you're always on the go, it's fine to replace those with a whey-protein shake you can carry with you in a flask.

This plan is paleo-based because you can't go far wrong with a Palaeolithic diet. It's anti-inflammatory, it's amazing for people with autoimmune issues, and there are so many delicious meal and snack options.

There are also a few nice surprises mixed in with the evening meals, because I want you to see that it's definitely not a restrictive plan that means you can't enjoy the things you love. I certainly do. There are thousands upon thousands of amazing paleo recipes out there. I'm an 'experimental' cook, I throw it all in and hope for the best, hence I'm not including recipes and claiming to be some kind of expert, but there are plenty of unbelievable paleo chefs out there if you'd feel safer following a recipe.

If you're wondering why I'm getting you to do lunges after lunch, it's because you're activating the biggest muscle group in your body without even have to put a pair of leggings on. By activating those muscle groups, your body will instantly level out your insulin levels, to stop you storing any sugar as fat. It will get your body into the habit of utilising any sugars you've consumed. You can also have apple cider vinegar before each meal. It's up to you. As you've probably realised, I'm an all-or-nothing kind of girl, so of course I do both.

Finally, I think it's so important for me to say this. If you have a wobble and have a doughnut, all is not lost. Have some activated charcoal or have a nice organic detox tea, and crack on. This is not all or nothing, so you don't have to go back to the beginning, just pick up where you left off.

# Your small but perfectly formed reset shopping list

I'm not going to give you a crazily long list of things to buy and demand you own a sauna, spike mat and blue blocking glasses before you begin the two-week reset because that's ridiculous. I always wanted this plan to be accessible.

The only things I would recommend you should buy, if and when you can, are the products listed below, which I have found to be incredibly beneficial.

However, I also want to say that if you don't use them all it's totally fine and it doesn't mean the plan won't work. It's up to you what feels right.

- Digestive enzymes

- MCT oil or powder

- Bone-broth powder

- Electrolyte powder

- Molkosan

- Aloe vera

- Epsom salts

- Clipper organic Latin American instant coffee

- Matcha tea powder.

If you would like suggestions of good places to buy products, please see the section at the back of the book for companies I trust and would happily recommend.

I don't have any affiliation with them or earn money if you buy from them, but I have worked with them all, so I know how good they are.

# *How to make MCT coffee*

Brew up some delicious coffee, add one tablespoon of MCT oil. Blend well and enjoy with one or two L-theanine tablets.

~

# *How to make Matcha tea*

Mix one tablespoon of Matcha powder with hot water. Add one to two tablespoons of MCT oil and whizz up, and serve with one or two L-theanine tablets!

~

## LET'S DO THIS!

I've created a chart for each day, with a suggestion for mood, food, movement and rest. This is a holistic plan that helps support your body and mind, so although I totally get that you may not be able to do everything each day, do try to take a balanced approach between all four categories.

Just focusing on food and exercise is honestly short-changing yourself and making things more difficult. Keep an open mind and you'll soon see how these little rituals, much as you may resist them at first, will make you feel amazing.

I find if I exercise in the morning, I don't have time to make excuses, so that's when I prefer to move. If you'd rather exercise later in the day, do what works for you. The timing is just a suggestion.

When it comes to rest, I've given four options throughout the plan. I like to use all of these tools, on alternate days, but you may find that you prefer one, or find it the most effective. Feel free to just stick to Epsom salt baths if that's your favourite: no need to invest in spike mats or infra-red saunas.

I recommend taking Molkosan and aloe vera first thing if you feel bloated and have gut issues. Feel free to skip this if you don't have any problems with your digestion. Take 1 capful of Molkosan and up to three caps of aloe vera, mixed in a large glass of water.

# WEEK ONE: **DAY 1**

## FIRST THING

**MOOD:**
Have a hot shower, then turn the temperature to cold for 10–20 seconds. Blast the water on the top of your spine to help with hormone balancing and to stimulate the vagus nerve.

**FOOD:**
Molkosan and aloe vera in water.

**MOVEMENT:** 20 minutes:
Slow walk and focus on breathing
*or* fast walk listening to up-tempo music
*or* jog to music – run for the chorus and walk for the verse.

## BREAKFAST

**FOOD:**
1 glass of water with electrolytes.
MCT coffee *or* Matcha tea (see page 215 for recipes).

## MID-MORNING

**FOOD:** Three eggs, scrambled, with cheese. MCT coffee *or* protein shake if out and about.

## LUNCH (BETWEEN 12 NOON AND 2 P.M.)

**FOOD:**
Tablespoon of apple cider vinegar in a glass of water, followed by chicken mayo salad on sourdough.

**MOVEMENT:**
Immediately after eating, do 10 lunges on each leg.

## SNACK (OPTIONAL)

**FOOD:** Kombucha *or* MCT coffee *or* Matcha tea.

## DINNER

**FOOD:** Steak with rocket and mushrooms, followed by a cheese plate and sourdough.

## EVENING

**FOOD:** Molkosan and aloe vera in water.

**REST:**
20-minute hot Epsom salt bath. Finish with a cold shower
*or* Wim Hof breathing exercise *or* a sauna *or* lie on a spike mat.

# WEEK ONE: **DAY 2**

## FIRST THING

### MOOD:
Hot shower, then turn temperature to cold for 10–20 seconds on top of your spine to help with hormone balancing/stimulate the vagus nerve.

### FOOD:
Molkosan and aloe vera in water.

### MOVEMENT:
20 minutes: choose from day-one options.

## BREAKFAST

### FOOD:
1 glass of water with electrolytes. MCT coffee *or* Matcha tea.

## MID-MORNING

### FOOD:
Kombucha *or* MCT coffee *or* Matcha tea *or* bone broth with MCT.

## LUNCH (BETWEEN 12 NOON AND 2 P.M.)

### FOOD:
Digestive enzyme.
Smoked salmon with avocado and eggs, cooked however you like them.

### MOVEMENT:
Immediately after eating, do 10 lunges on each leg.

## SNACK (OPTIONAL)

FOOD: Kombucha *or* MCT coffee *or* Matcha tea.

## DINNER

### FOOD:
Fish fried in butter with capers. Quinoa with garlic and chopped veg.
A few squares of dark chocolate with salt.

## EVENING

### REST:
20-minute hot Epsom salt bath. Finish with a cold shower
*or* Wim Hof breathing exercise *or* a sauna *or* lie on a spike mat.

# WEEK ONE: **DAY 3**

## FIRST THING

MOOD:
Hot shower, then turn temperature to cold for 10–20 seconds on top of your spine
to help with hormone balancing/stimulate the vagus nerve.

FOOD:
Molkosan and aloe
vera in water.

MOVEMENT:
20-minute walk and deep breathing
*or* a fast walk listening to up-tempo music
*or* a jog where you run for the chorus and walk for the verse
(all can be done at any time).

## BREAKFAST

FOOD:
1 glass of water with electrolytes. MCT coffee *or* Matcha tea.

## MID-MORNING

FOOD:
Kombucha *or* MCT coffee *or* Matcha tea *or* bone broth with MCT.

## LUNCH (BETWEEN 12 NOON AND 2 P.M.)

FOOD:
Organic whey protein.
Activated nuts (see page 240).

MOVEMENT:
Immediately after eating,
do 10 lunges on each leg.

## SNACK (OPTIONAL)

FOOD: Kombucha *or* MCT coffee *or* Matcha tea.

## DINNER

FOOD:
Chicken thighs cooked in organic stock. Mixed veg. White rice cooked in bone broth.
Dark chocolate.

## EVENING

REST:
20-minute hot Epsom salt bath. Finish with a cold shower
*or* Wim Hof breathing exercise *or* a sauna *or* lie on a spike mat.

# WEEK ONE: **DAY 4**

## FIRST THING

**MOOD:**
Hot shower, then turn temperature to cold for 10–20 seconds on top of your spine
to help with hormone balancing/stimulate the vagus nerve.

**FOOD:**
Molkosan and aloe
vera in water.

**MOVEMENT:**
20-minute walk and deep breathing
*or* a fast walk listening to up-tempo music
*or* a jog where you run for the chorus and walk for the verse
(all can be done at any time).

## BREAKFAST

**FOOD:**
1 glass of water with electrolytes.  MCT coffee  *or*  Matcha tea.

## MID-MORNING

**FOOD:**
Kombucha  *or*  MCT coffee  *or*  Matcha tea  *or*  bone broth with MCT.

## LUNCH (BETWEEN 12 NOON AND 2 P.M.)

**FOOD:**
Prawn with avocado, rocket, cucumber
and mayo on sourdough.

**MOVEMENT:**
Immediately after eating,
do 10 lunges on each leg.

## SNACK (OPTIONAL)

FOOD: Kombucha  *or*  MCT coffee  *or*  Matcha tea.

## DINNER

**FOOD:**
Lamb chops with mint and Greek salad.

## EVENING

**REST:**
20-minute hot Epsom salt bath. Finish with a cold shower
*or* Wim Hof breathing exercise  *or*  a sauna  *or*  lie on a spike mat.

# WEEK ONE: **DAY 5**

## FIRST THING

### MOOD:
Hot shower, then turn temperature to cold for 10–20 seconds on top of your spine to help with hormone balancing/stimulate the vagus nerve.

### FOOD:
Molkosan and aloe vera in water.

### MOVEMENT:
20-minute walk and deep breathing
*or* a fast walk listening to up-tempo music
*or* a jog where you run for the chorus and walk for the verse
(all can be done at any time).

## BREAKFAST

### FOOD:
1 glass of water with electrolytes. MCT coffee *or* Matcha tea.

## MID-MORNING

### FOOD:
Kombucha *or* MCT coffee *or* Matcha tea *or* bone broth with MCT.

## LUNCH (BETWEEN 12 NOON AND 2 P.M.)

### FOOD:
Extend your fast by blending bone broth with MCT oil.

### MOVEMENT:
Immediately after eating, do 10 lunges on each leg.

## SNACK (OPTIONAL)

FOOD: Kombucha *or* MCT coffee *or* Matcha tea.

## DINNER

### FOOD:
Sourdough pizza *or* any of the meat dishes from this week.
One glass of organic red wine.

## EVENING

### REST:
20-minute hot Epsom salt bath. Finish with a cold shower
*or* Wim Hof breathing exercise *or* a sauna *or* lie on a spike mat.

# WEEK ONE: **DAY 6**

## FIRST THING

### MOOD:
Hot shower, then turn temperature to cold for 10–20 seconds on top of your spine to help with hormone balancing/stimulate the vagus nerve.

### FOOD:
Molkosan and aloe vera in water.

### MOVEMENT:
20-minute walk and deep breathing
*or* a fast walk listening to up-tempo music
*or* a jog where you run for the chorus and walk for the verse
(all can be done at any time).

## BREAKFAST

### FOOD:
1 glass of water with electrolytes. MCT coffee *or* Matcha tea.

## MID-MORNING

### FOOD:
Kombucha *or* MCT coffee *or* Matcha tea *or* bone broth with MCT.

## LUNCH (BETWEEN 12 NOON AND 2 P.M.)

### FOOD:
Extend your fast by blending bone broth with MCT oil.

### MOVEMENT:
Immediately after eating, do 10 lunges on each leg.

## SNACK (OPTIONAL)

FOOD: Kombucha *or* MCT coffee *or* Matcha tea.

## DINNER

### FOOD:
Prawn and rice stir fry. Cook the rice using the bone broth.

## EVENING

### REST:
20-minute hot Epsom salt bath. Finish with a cold shower
*or* Wim Hof breathing exercise *or* a sauna *or* lie on a spike mat.

# WEEK ONE: **DAY 7**

## FIRST THING

**MOOD:**
Hot shower, then turn temperature to cold for 10–20 seconds on top of your spine
to help with hormone balancing/stimulate the vagus nerve.

**FOOD:**
Molkosan and aloe
vera in water.

**MOVEMENT:**
20-minute walk and deep breathing
*or* a fast walk listening to up-tempo music
*or* a jog where you run for the chorus and walk for the verse
(all can be done at any time).

## BREAKFAST

**FOOD:**
1 glass of water with electrolytes. MCT coffee *or* Matcha tea.

## MID-MORNING

**FOOD:**
Kombucha *or* MCT coffee *or* Matcha tea *or* bone broth with MCT.

## LUNCH (BETWEEN 12 NOON AND 2 P.M.)

**FOOD:**
Extend your fast by blending
bone broth with MCT oil.

**MOVEMENT:**
Immediately after eating,
do 10 lunges on each leg.

## SNACK (OPTIONAL)

**FOOD:** Kombucha *or* MCT coffee *or* Matcha tea.

## DINNER

**FOOD:**
Choose from any of the dinners from this week.

## EVENING

**REST:**
20-minute hot Epsom salt bath. Finish with a cold shower
*or* Wim Hof breathing exercise *or* a sauna *or* lie on a spike mat.

## WEEK TWO

This is where things ramp up, but don't put yourself under any pressure to increase the pace if you're not feeling ready. If you found week one a bit of a struggle, there's no shame in repeating it several times until you feel like it's time to take things to the next level.

You could repeat the first week for three weeks and then do week two for the fourth week so you've completed a month. Or make it a six-week plan and do three weeks of each.

It goes without saying that the more you push yourself, the quicker you'll get results. But if it takes you a bit longer to get there, it really doesn't matter. This is about you and no one else.

During this week we are increasing our fasting, and that means we are increasing autophagy, and helping to clean out our bodies. Also, we are not eating biscuits all day, which helps.

Feel free to mix and match the dinners in the second week if there's something you really love/don't really love.

# WEEK TWO: **DAY 8**

## FIRST THING

MOOD:
Hot shower, then turn temperature to cold for 30 seconds. Yes, you can!
Bonus points for putting your head under the cold water.

FOOD:
Molkosan and aloe
vera in water.

MOVEMENT:
20 minutes. Step it up this week.
Fast walk listening to up-tempo music
*or* jog where you run for the chorus and walk for the verse.

## BREAKFAST

FOOD:
1 glass of water with electrolytes. MCT coffee *or* Matcha tea.

## MID-MORNING

—

## LUNCH (BETWEEN 12 NOON AND 2 P.M.)

FOOD:
Full English breakfast
with sourdough.

MOVEMENT:
Immediately after eating,
do 15 lunges on each leg.

## SNACK

FOOD: Kombucha *and/or* herbal tea.

## DINNER

FOOD:
A roast with veg but no potatoes,
followed by cheese and a few squares of dark chocolate.

## EVENING

REST:
20-minute hot Epsom salt bath. Finish with a cold shower
*or* Wim Hof breathing exercise *or* a sauna *or* lie on a spike mat

# WEEK TWO: **DAY 9**

## FIRST THING

MOOD:
Hot shower, then turn temperature to cold for 30 seconds. Yes, you can!
Bonus points for putting your head under the cold water.

FOOD:
Molkosan and aloe
vera in water.

MOVEMENT:
20 minutes: fast walk listening to up-tempo music
*or* jog where you run for the chorus and walk for the verse.

## BREAKFAST

FOOD:
1 glass of water with electrolytes.  MCT coffee  *or*  Matcha tea.

## MID-MORNING

–

## LUNCH (BETWEEN 12 NOON AND 2 P.M.)

FOOD:
Two eggs, scrambled, with smoked salmon.

## SNACK

–

## DINNER

FOOD:
Leftover roast meat from Day 8, with salad and olive oil dressing.

## EVENING

REST:
20-minute hot Epsom salt bath. Finish with a cold shower
*or* Wim Hof breathing exercise  *or*  a sauna  *or*  lie on a spike mat.

# WEEK TWO: **DAY 10**

## FIRST THING

MOOD:
Hot shower, then turn temperature to cold for 30 seconds. Yes, you can!
Bonus points for putting your head under the cold water.

FOOD:
Molkosan and aloe
vera in water.

MOVEMENT:
20 minutes: fast walk listening to up-tempo music
or jog where you run for the chorus and walk for the verse.

## BREAKFAST

FOOD:
1 glass of water with electrolytes.  MCT coffee  or  Matcha tea.

## MID-MORNING

—

## LUNCH (BETWEEN 12 NOON AND 2 P.M.)

FOOD:
Bone broth, eggs, smoked salmon,
avocado and kombucha.

MOVEMENT:
Immediately after eating,
do 15 lunges on each leg.

## SNACK (OPTIONAL)

FOOD:  MCT coffee  or  bone broth with MCT.

## DINNER

FOOD:
Baked chicken thighs (skin on!) with a goat's cheese salad and quinoa.

## EVENING

REST:
20-minute hot Epsom salt bath. Finish with a cold shower
or  Wim Hof breathing exercise  or  a sauna  or  lie on a spike mat.

# WEEK TWO: **DAY 11**

## FIRST THING

### MOOD:
Hot shower, then turn temperature to cold for 30 seconds. Yes, you can!
Bonus points for putting your head under the cold water.

### FOOD:
Molkosan and aloe vera in water.

### MOVEMENT:
20 minutes: fast walk listening to up-tempo music
*or* jog where you run for the chorus and walk for the verse.

## BREAKFAST

### FOOD:
1 glass of water with electrolytes. MCT coffee *or* Matcha tea *or* Rooibos tea.

## MID-MORNING

FOOD: MCT coffee *or* Matcha tea *or* Rooibos tea.

## LUNCH (BETWEEN 12 NOON AND 2 P.M.)

FOOD: Kombucha.

## SNACK

FOOD: Celery juice *and/or* bone broth.

## DINNER

### FOOD:
Bone broth soup
with sandwich made with sourdough,
outdoor-bred ham or organic chicken and
grass-fed butter.
Chia pudding with coconut milk and vanilla.

### MOVEMENT:
Immediately after eating,
do 15 lunges on each leg.

## EVENING

### REST:
20-minute hot Epsom salt bath. Finish with a cold shower
*or* Wim Hof breathing exercise *or* a sauna *or* lie on a spike mat.

# WEEK TWO: **DAY 12**

## FIRST THING

**MOOD:**
Hot shower, then turn temperature to cold for 30 seconds. Yes, you can!
Bonus points for putting your head under the cold water.

**FOOD:**
Molkosan and aloe vera in water.

**MOVEMENT:**
20 minutes: fast walk listening to up-tempo music
*or* jog where you run for the chorus and walk for the verse.

## BREAKFAST

**FOOD:**
1 glass of water with electrolytes. MCT coffee *or* Matcha tea *or* Rooibos tea.

## MID-MORNING

**FOOD:** MCT coffee *or* Matcha tea *or* Rooibos tea.

## LUNCH (BETWEEN 12 NOON AND 2 P.M.)

**FOOD:** Kombucha.

## SNACK

**FOOD:** Celery juice *and/or* bone broth.

## DINNER

**FOOD:**
Garlic prawn salad.
A few squares of dark chocolate.
Cheese.

**MOVEMENT:**
Immediately after eating,
do 15 lunges on each leg.

## EVENING

**REST:**
20-minute hot Epsom salt bath. Finish with a cold shower
*or* Wim Hof breathing exercise *or* a sauna *or* lie on a spike mat.

# WEEK TWO: **DAY 13**

## FIRST THING

**MOOD:**
Hot shower, then turn temperature to cold for 30 seconds. Yes, you can!
Bonus points for putting your head under the cold water.

**FOOD:**
Molkosan and aloe vera in water.

**MOVEMENT:**
20 minutes: fast walk listening to up-tempo music
*or* jog where you run for the chorus and walk for the verse.

## BREAKFAST

**FOOD:**
1 glass of water with electrolytes. MCT coffee *or* Matcha tea *or* Rooibos tea.

## MID-MORNING

**FOOD:** MCT coffee *or* Matcha tea *or* Rooibos tea.

## LUNCH (BETWEEN 12 NOON AND 2 P.M.)

**FOOD:** Kombucha.

## SNACK

**FOOD:** Celery juice *and/or* bone broth.

## DINNER

**FOOD:**
Steak with chips air-fried in avocado oil.
If you don't have an air fryer, oven-cook using
avocado oil.

**MOVEMENT:**
Immediately after eating,
do 15 lunges on each leg.

## EVENING

**REST:**
20-minute hot Epsom salt bath. Finish with a cold shower
*or* Wim Hof breathing exercise *or* a sauna *or* lie on a spike mat.

# WEEK TWO: **DAY 14**

## FIRST THING

MOOD:
Hot shower, then turn temperature to cold for 30 seconds. Yes, you can!
Bonus points for putting your head under the cold water.

FOOD:
Molkosan and aloe
vera in water.

MOVEMENT:
20 minutes: fast walk listening to up-tempo music
*or* jog where you run for the chorus and walk for the verse.

## BREAKFAST

FOOD:
1 glass of water with electrolytes. MCT coffee *or* Matcha tea *or* Rooibos tea.

## MID-MORNING

FOOD: MCT coffee *or* Matcha tea *or* Rooibos tea.

## LUNCH (BETWEEN 12 NOON AND 2 P.M.)

FOOD: Kombucha.

## SNACK

FOOD: Celery juice *and/or* bone broth.

## DINNER

FOOD:
*You've done it!*
Reward yourself with a Full English with
sourdough, a glass of organic red wine
and a few squares of dark chocolate.

MOVEMENT:
Immediately after eating,
do 15 lunges on each leg.

## EVENING

REST:
20-minute hot Epsom salt bath. Finish with a cold shower
*or* Wim Hof breathing exercise *or* a sauna *or* lie on a spike mat.

If you completed the two-week reset, please give yourself a massive pat on the back. And if you stumbled a little here and there? Who cares? Dust yourself off and try again!

# APPENDIX I

# SUPERMARKET-FRIENDLY SHOPPING LISTS

As a busy mum, I generally buy about 80 per cent of my food from regular supermarkets and the rest from farmers' markets, online and the occasional health store. So I've based my suggestions on what I can find at my local supermarket, to keep this as accessible as possible.

What I want to show you with these shopping lists is that it is easy to embark on a nutritious lifestyle. You don't have to seek out weird superfoods or exotic berries to feel good and get lean. You just need to eat real food to take you out of the peaks and troughs of cravings for junk.

These lists contain easy-to-find fresh produce to help you with your weekly or monthly shopping trip. With these ingredients as the basis for your meals, you'll know that you're getting a wide variety of vitamins, minerals and nutrients to feed your body, and importantly, your brain.

Get online and seek out recipes for paleo diets that use your favourite ingredients. There are so many great chefs out there, and cooking doesn't need to be complicated. One meal that my kids love is just a tray of organic chicken wings, baked in the oven until crispy. How simple is that?

Nowadays I buy a lot of my meat online rather than from supermarkets, as my priority is outdoor-reared high-welfare meat, and that is not always easy to find on the chiller shelves. It also cuts out the middleman and gives the money directly to the farmer. I've suggested some of my preferred online meat suppliers at the back of the book.

For me, buying organic is important, but let's be clear: it's not everything. If organic food feels out of reach for you, don't worry about it. Just stick to keeping as close to the natural food as possible, and you'll be doing brilliantly. We are lucky in the UK to have some of the best farming practices in the world, so if you can't buy organic, buy British.

By no means do you have to buy everything on this list! Just pick and choose what you like and what you can work with for yourself and your family.

## Beef

I always buy British beef. My preference is to buy from smaller farms, as I want to avoid the antibiotics and hormones in factory-farmed meat. It needs to be grass-fed both for the welfare of the animal and for the best nutrition, and I prefer organic, but like I said above, don't get too hung up on this.

- Beef steak mince
- Beef liver
- Diced beef
- Beef casserole steak
- Beef carvery joint
- Beef brisket

## Chicken

I generally try and buy chicken on the bone because I will re-use the bones in making bone broth and also it makes the meat tastier. As before, I prioritise free range and organic.

- Whole chicken
- Chicken thigh fillets
- Chicken drumsticks
- Chicken liver

## Lamb

As I said earlier in the book, lamb is generally reared outdoors, which makes it grass-fed, so you don't have to pay the organic price tag for this. However, I like to support that industry, so I prefer to buy organic where I can.

- Lamb mince
- Lamb diced leg
- Lamb stewing
- Lamb neck

## Pork

The pork industry has some of the most abhorrent farming conditions. I do not endorse eating pork from factory farms, not just because they are cruel, but because the nutrition of an outdoor-reared animal is superior. Please pay attention to where your meat is coming from and support local farms where you can. Outdoor-reared is essential for pork.

- Pork loin steaks
- Pork leg

- Pork shoulder joint
- Streaky bacon
- Sausages (minimum meat content 85 per cent and watch out for grains, oils and fillers)

## Turkey

I'm noticing more and more outdoor-bred turkey in the freezer department, which I love to see. It's a great meat to use and if it is organic, which mine always is, make sure you utilise that fat.

- Turkey breast mince
- Turkey breast steaks
- Turkey diced breast
- Turkey diced thighs

## Venison

- Venison steaks and mince

## Fish

Aim for a portion of oily fish at least three times a week. The omega-3 fatty acids in fish are powerful contributors to brain function. Studies suggest eating oily fish can help with brain fog, as well as being useful for children with ADHD.

I've started to order from online fish markets, again cutting out the middleman, and supporting our local fisheries instead of farms in the Far East. It gets delivered to my door frozen.

- Wild-caught smoked salmon (avoid farmed salmon)
- Wild-caught or North Atlantic/Alaskan salmon steaks or fillets (you'll see these are a totally different colour from

farmed salmon, because of their natural diet)

- Fresh and smoked mackerel
- Wild-caught frozen cod fillets
- Sardine fillets in brine or olive oil (avoid the ones in sunflower oil)

## Seafood

- Atlantic wild-caught prawns
- Live mussels
- Scallops
- Wild-caught frozen squid
- Wild-caught lobster
- Wild-caught crab

As long as all of these are from the UK, I wouldn't be so vigilant about the farming methods: just get the nutrition.

## Eggs

For me, it's really important to buy organic, free-range eggs, but I get that these are expensive. Eggs are a total superfood, full of protein and good fats. If you can't buy organic, you're still eating something that's incredibly good for you. Just do your best.

- Mixed-size organic eggs
- Liquid egg whites (free range)
- Quails eggs (free to fly)

## Dairy

I don't eat a ton of dairy, but I don't avoid it either. In fact, I'm getting quite into whole milk, and the kids love it. As with everything I eat, when it comes to dairy I'm looking for food as close to its natural state as possible. So that means cheese with no artificial colours or other additives. Any cheese that has been fermented is going to give your gut some great bacteria, so Tim Spector is a fan of them for the health of your microbiome. And dairy is a great source of fat and protein.

My preference is dairy from grass-fed, organic cows, as factory-farm-produced animals are fed a lot of antibiotics and hormones which end up in their milk.

- Whole milk
- Full-fat yogurt with no added sugar or sweetener
- Parmesan
- Cheddar
- Mozzarella
- Feta

## Vegetables

Again, I try to go for organic when it comes to vegetables. I smother all our vegetables in Maldon sea salt and grass-fed butter – your body needs fat to absorb all the vitamins in the vegetables.

Personally, other than an occasional celery juice, I don't recommend juicing your vegetables, as you lose the fibre and the juices can be hard to digest.

STARCHY

- Beetroot
- Butternut squash
- Carrots
- Parsnips
- Baby potatoes (organic)
- Sweet potatoes (organic)
- White potatoes (organic)

NON-STARCHY

- Avocado
- Red onion
- White onion
- Sweet peppers
- Spring onions
- Rocket
- Leeks
- Garlic
- Courgettes
- Celery
- Broccoli

## Fruit

- Strawberries, organic
- Blueberries, organic (otherwise wash thoroughly before eating)
- Bananas
- Pears
- Melons
- Grapefruit
- Apples
- Dates

## Oils

I'm really into the health benefits of extra virgin olive oil, and have discovered that you get the maximum health benefits if the oil was harvested no more than twelve months ago. This can be hard to find in the supermarket, but there are some great online suppliers, and I've given some of these at the back of the book.

- Extra-virgin olive oil in a dark bottle (to avoid it being damaged by light)
- Coconut oil organic
- Grass-fed butter
- Avocado oil
- Organic lard or tallow

## Nuts and seeds

Nuts are amazing for mood and brain health. I like to 'activate' nuts, which makes them easier to digest, and easier for the body to absorb the nutrients. If you'd like to try this, soak nuts overnight in cold water and a pinch of sea salt, then drain and dry, and bake them in a cool oven at 70° for at least eight hours. If you like a sweeter treat, you can add some honey or maple syrup to the nuts before you bake them. However, this makes them extremely moreish, so be warned!

- Almonds
- Almond butter
- Pumpkin seeds
- Chia seeds
- Brazil nuts
- Mixed nuts
- Tahini

## Bread

The only bread I personally eat is sourdough. The fermentation process of sourdough helps to break down that gluten molecule, hence less bloating and I find the longer it's fermented, the less my bloat! If you can find forty-eight-hour fermented sourdough, that's the best, otherwise opt for white sourdough over brown as the wholegrain variety can irritate your gut, which defeats the whole point!

## Flours

If you're going to be brave and make your own sourdough, make sure you're using organic flour.

Otherwise, I don't particularly buy flours, other than some almond flour occasionally, though it's pretty expensive.

If you use flour for cooking, such as for coating chicken before baking it, I like to use arrowroot with some mixed herbs and garlic powder rather than flour. Just dip the chicken into beaten egg, then into the arrowroot mixture, and bake in the oven for a homemade KFC.

## Condiments

Avoid all condiments that contain added sugar and vegetable oil. The only companies that I recommend for sugar-free and vegetable-oil-free condiments are Hunter and Gather and some Stokes products. These are available in most large supermarkets and online.

# APPENDIX II

# MY RECOMMENDED SUPPLIERS

I feel like I'm constantly learning about nutrition, and finding amazing new companies who are creating products that cater to the healthy lifestyle I'm working on. So this list of favourite suppliers changes all the time, and I always share my latest discoveries over on Instagram (@daviniataylor). You can also visit my website at www.willpowders.com for more products.

### Protein powders

https://theorganicproteincompany.co.uk/
https://www.bulk.com/uk/
https://amazinggrasscompany.co.uk/?redirect=region

### Collagen

https://reviveactive.com/
https://www.pureagen.com/
https://www.planetpaleo.co/
https://hunterandgatherfoods.com

## Bone broth

https://www.planetpaleo.co/
https://www.ossaorganic.com/

## Nootropics

https://troscriptions.com/
https://www.naturalstacks.com
https://www.functionalself.co.uk/
https://www.onnit.com/
www.onnorlife.com

## Supplements

https://thedrug.store
https://www.allergyresearchgroup.com
https://getkion.com/
https://www.highernature
uk.thorne.com

## Wellbeing and nutrition

https://www.wellgevity.com
https://www.pippacampbellhealth.com
https://bengreenfieldfitness.com/

## Health testing

www.omnos.me
www.lifecodegx.com

## Beauty

www.jasonnaturalcare.co.uk

www.mariereynoldslondon.com

www.thedecree.com

www.neostrata.com

www.facemattersskincare.com

## Food and drinks

www.plenishdrinks.com

www.coombefarmorganic.co.uk

www.daylesford.com

helenbrowningsorganic.co.uk

biona.co.uk

shop.meridianfoods.co.uk/online/shop

www.stokessauces.co.uk
   (check for sunflower oil in some of their sauces)

www.gokombucha.co.uk

equinoxkombucha.com

# ACKNOWLEDGEMENTS

The first person I would like to thank has to be Becca Barr, my agent, who convinced me I could get a book deal and finally make orderly sense of my exploits in self-experimentation for others to learn from or in some cases avoid! Then follows my gratitude to Pippa Wright at Orion Spring for giving me the opportunity to become a published author and Jordan Paramor for her patience and brilliance working with me by putting pen to paper. And of course the people who, unlike me, took the time to study, to actually go to university, read books, sit in lectures, revise like mad, share their knowledge and constantly invest in their education from who I have learned so much, including Dr Tamsin Lewis, Professor Tim Spector, Pippa Campbell, Dave Asprey, Tim Grey, Dr Cate Shannon, Dr Rachel Gow and Dr Tommy Wood to name but a few!

Lovingly, always by my side on the ride, are The Them, my crew of middle-aged misfits, and of course my kids for constantly pushing my buttons, challenging and loving me unconditionally in equal measure! Lastly there is, of course, my ever-supportive husband and best friend Matthew who generally gets the raw deal with my failures and life downturns but is always there with a smile to pick up the pieces ... behind every successful book is an extremely strong partner with the patience of a saint! Thank you for your faith, Matthew, and instilling confidence in me, as so many times in this rollercoaster I've lacked so much.

Actress, fitness fanatic and health biohacker extraordinaire, Davinia Taylor's career began as an actress and television presenter.

Davinia's heavily documented party lifestyle led to a dependency on alcohol, post-natal depression and a struggle to regain her pre-baby body after four children. But, after genetic testing, Davinia biohacked her way to optimum health, losing nearly three stone in six months, and keeping it off. She shares her story through public events and on her rapidly growing Instagram (@daviniataylor). You can visit her website at www.willpowders.com